The **FATHER FIGURE** of **FITNESS**

Steve Thomas BSc (Hons)
Sport Scientist

The **FATHER FIGURE** of **FITNESS**

First published in the UK in 2023

Published by G2 Entertainment

www.g2books.co.uk

© Steve Thomas 2023

All rights reserved. No part of this work may be reproduced or utilised in any form or by any means, electronic or mechanical, including photocopying, recording or by any information storage and retrieval system, without prior written permission of the publisher.

Printed and bound in the UK

ISBN 978-1-78281-846-5

The views in this book are those of the author but they are general views only and readers are urged to consult the relevant and qualified specialist for individual advice in particular situations.

G2 Entertainment hereby exclude all liability to the extent permitted by law of any errors or omissions in this book and for any loss, damage or expense (whether direct or indirect) suffered by a third party relying on any information contained in this book.

All our best endeavours have been made to secure copyright clearance for every photograph used but in the event of any copyright owner being overlooked please address correspondence to G2 Entertainment, Unit 16a Beaufort Road, Reigate, Surrey, RH2 9DJ.

All images in this book are copyright and have been provided courtesy of the following:

WIKICOMMONS
commons.wikimedia.org

SHUTTERSTOCK
www.shutterstock.com

STEVE THOMAS

Design & Artwork: ALEX YOUNG

Publisher: JULES GAMMOND

Written by: STEVE THOMAS

Contents

1) Introduction 04
  – A brief personal introduction
  – Personal endorsements
  – Motivation for writing this book

2) Personal background 07
  – The start of my journey
  – My sporting background

3) Myths and misconceptions 12
  – Forty of the most common myths and misconceptions

4) The missing link – human biomechanics 22
  – The gait cycle – understanding how we all move
  – The human spine; why the world is full of back pain

5) Leg Length discrepancy 32
  – Its importance and how to measure it

6) Skeletal compensation leads to injury 39
  – We are all getting worse, not better
  – Medical statistics

7) Movement analysis 41
  – The key to everyone's success
  – The human kinetic chain of movement
  – Examples of the human kinetic chain

8) Development of my 100,000 system 67
  – How my method has evolved
  – The 30 key components

9) Summary 152
  – Exercise spreadsheet
  – Example of a training routine

10) My top tips 174
  – Ten Golden Rules for your success

11) Conclusion 178

Introduction

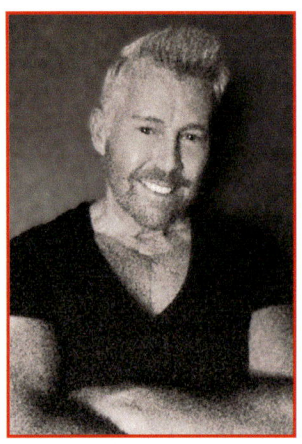

My name is Steve Thomas.

I have a Bachelor of Science degree in Sport Science and I have been an Elite Personal Trainer for over 37 years. I introduced personal training to the UK in the mid- to late 1980s, and my aim, my goal, my ambition and my motivation were to introduce scientific knowledge into all aspects and forms of fitness, exercise and sport. Progressing from grassroots beginner level to working with some of the world's elite athletes, I have amassed more than 100,000 one-to-one professional personal training sessions during those 37 years.

During this time the exercise and fitness industry has been **booming**. Growing from the uncertain, hesitant and humble beginnings of the aerobics classes and Jane Fonda workouts of the 1980s, it has exploded into a $100 billion, global industry and exercise and fitness have become the *holy grail* for those seeking physical and mental wellbeing.

There now exists a plethora of exercising choices – walking, jogging, running, rowing, stepping, boxing, cross-fit, circuit training, weight training, HIIT (high-intensity interval training), spinning classes, Pilates, yoga, water aerobics, skipping, swimming, stretching, tai chi, qigong, martial arts, plyometric training, zumba, bootcamp training, military training, kickboxing, pole fitness, barre fitness, hula fit, aerial hoop, trampolining, body combat and more.

With hundreds of millions of dedicated exercising disciples around the world, health and fitness has become a benchmark for social change. It stands for success and achievement, and personal trainers have become an essential 'fashion' accessory, for those who strive for self-improvement exude an aura of prosperity and authority.

Exercising has become a very, very important subject and part of many individuals'

INTRODUCTION

everyday life, with everyone searching for the best methods, routines and regimes. But do we **really understand** what exercise choices to make?

As a **sport scientist** and having worked with many of the UK's top medical specialists and a catalogue of the rich and famous, I have always seen things differently and I have always done things differently.

> "The father figure of fitness, Steve is a professional, elite exercise specialist and a true visionary – simply the best."
> Earl of Snowdon, King Charles III's cousin.

> "Steve's deep insight and knowledge of the human body are masterful – the best personal trainer I have ever had."
> Lady Alexander of Weedon.

> "Steve is without doubt the best in the business."
> Alan Watson MCSP.HPC, leading UK physiotherapist.

> "Steve's knowledge, experience and professionalism makes him unparalleled in his field."
> Clive D Lathey, DO MSc Sports Medicine, leading UK osteopath and sports injury specialist.

> "Steve trained me for 20 years. For anyone to become such an important part of your life for so long says it all. Making exercise second nature is a huge talent. Thank you so much."
> Leanda von Halle.

> **"Quite simply the WORLD'S BEST PERSONAL TRAINER."**
> C. Delevingne.

INTRODUCTION

My background, education and experience have afforded me a unique perspective of the evolution of fitness and exercise, and this is why I have felt a duty, a necessity, to put pen to paper and write this book. It's a book that may ruffle feathers and may even be judged as controversial, but it's a book that is needed at this time.

As a professional exercise specialist, I am going to explain why everyone is getting it wrong. YES, EVERYONE IS GETTING IT WRONG. It is 2023, and an endless variety of exercising options is available to each and every one of us – **but you have been forgotten**. My job, my career, my objectives, and my sole motivation have been all about making **your exercise all about you**.

We need a fundamental shift in our approach to exercising, a sea change in our understanding of how and why to make certain exercise choices and decisions. It's time to forget everything you have been taught and start again.

It's time to restart *your* education in exercise.

This book, my methods, my systems and programmes are *not* controversial. In a world where everyone knows and accepts that exercising is unquestionably a good thing to do, it is a forthright and honest critique of where we are in the evolution of exercising. Everything I advocate is based on medical science and 37 years of practical one-to-one experience. I have developed my 100,000 exercise system to be **unique and the most comprehensive exercise system ever formulated**.

This system has been designed especially for **you**. Follow my routines and it will change the way you think about exercising and the way you train for ever.

If you want to continue being stuck in a rut and out of date, just following trends, then this book is not for you. If you want to be at the cutting edge of the latest scientific and medical tips, techniques, ideas and exercise programmes, and understand the fundamental foundations that your exercising must be based on, then please read on.

Whatever your goals or ambitions, let me be your personal trainer. Let my knowledge and experience guide you towards achieving more efficient results faster.

This book is written from the heart. It is written to give back to an industry that has given me a wonderful career, but it is mainly written for **you**. Please enjoy it.

Personal background

The start of my journey.

Having been a sports-mad youngster, it was almost inevitable that I would seek out an academic degree course that would reflect this obsessive interest. My **sport science** degree was intense and highly scientific, but it delivered a comprehensive knowledge of the internal and external workings of the human body. The initial euphoria of gaining my Bachelor of Science degree was quickly tempered by the sobering realisation that no one in the outside world had ever heard of **sport science**, let alone understood what it meant.

This was daunting and frustrating. I believed that the scientific knowledge I had accumulated over the years would be very beneficial to the multitudes involved in sports, health and exercise, and I was determined after years of blood, sweat, toil and tears to change the world and introduce science into the world of exercise and fitness.

I had learned how the body is put together: its anatomy, its highly complex musculoskeletal system, how it moved, the immense forces it absorbs, the compensatory capabilities, the intricate millisecond timings of complex motor skills, the unbelievably efficient cardiovascular network, delivering blood flow with mind-blowing precision, the incredible cardiorespiratory system, exchanging gases automatically with computerised timing. And then there was the human brain, the control tower that orders and orchestrates the symphony of every psychological, every neurological and every physiological command.

I had gained a true understanding of how we stand, walk, jog, run, sprint, jump, twist, rotate, lift, bend and push. I understood the physical and physiological demands of every golf swing, every tennis serve, every rugby tackle, every slam dunk, every somersault, every press-up and every squat. More importantly, I was a **specialist in exercise prescription**.

As a newly fledged sport scientist, I moved to London to confront the fitness industry head-on. In the mid-1980s, the fitness industry barely existed, and I quickly learned that exercise, activities and sports were controlled, organised,

PERSONAL BACKGROUND

managed and coached by people who were out of date, in a time warp and blinkered, using methodologies and training principles that hadn't been updated for decades. They were using hand-me-down knowledge from past generations of ex-players, professionals and coaches. There was no real scientific or medical understanding of the human body; there was even a real resistance to any new exercise science.

I knew this had to change. I knew I had to break down these stubborn barriers to change. I knew I had to find a way to educate and prove that I had something different and special to offer.

An understanding of the history of exercise demonstrated that any new exercise ideas were mainly 'one size fits all', group-based training like high- or low-impact aerobics, jazzercise, step aerobics or circuit training. It was clear that despite the growing number of exercise methods, programmes and principles and the existing trend for group training, the general population had never been so physically sedentary.

Computers and mobile phones were just starting to have their effect. Everyone was out of shape, full of back pain, lacking in motivation and interest. Exercising regularly had become a chore not a pleasure, and the abundant exercise choices were confusing. Nobody really knew what the best routines or regimes would be for them. Should they walk, jog, run, lift weights, cycle, swim or sign up for group classes?

It was quite clear to me that the whole exercising world was guessing. It had lost clarity and simplicity. We had been searching for the perfect one-system-fits-all approach but it was getting too complex and simply wasn't working. We had lost sight of who and what we are – human beings with amazing human bodies that were out of kilter. We were individuals needing individual approaches and different mindsets. Now was the time for me to strike.

By chance, the wife of a very famous person rang me and suggested that I become a personal trainer for her husband. I had never before heard those two very simple words placed together, and the request gave me the lightbulb moment I was searching for – my vehicle for incorporating not only science but also a much-needed personal element into every individual's training.

The individual in question had significant back pain. I set about remodelling his exercise programme and, steadily but surely, he responded. He was delighted, and I was exuberant, as this was the true start of my personal training career.

PERSONAL BACKGROUND

Personal training really fed the need for service and personal attention; it was something different, progressive and unique. I was able to use my sport science knowledge to create something that was utterly individual and uniquely personal.

I understood how and why the human body could move with grace, fluidity and symmetry, but more importantly, I could recognise acutely the signs and symptoms that resulted when this human chain of actions and reactions faltered; when it deviated from its slick, well-oiled, majestic flow.

Throughout the next 37 years I worked tirelessly with thousands of individuals, completing my apprenticeship and earning my stripes. Moulding my methods, experimenting and trying all options, ideas, routines and regimes old and new, I monitored closely how different clients reacted physically and mentally to the various strategies I employed. The whole world of fitness was starting to **boom**.

I fully understand that during a *boom* in any industry there will be a bombardment of ideas, advice, suggestions and opinions that flood the market and come from a variety of sources – some good, some bad, some considered, some not and some completely ridiculous. The exercise/fitness world has certainly succumbed to this phenomenon.

Since the explosion in interest in exercise from the 1980s onwards, many voices have put forward their mantras for consumption by the masses as everybody strives to find their way, searching for the best advice, experimenting and testing out each theory along the way.

This inevitably leads to vastly different and conflicting opinions, confusion of ideas and advice and misinterpretation and misrepresentation of information and advice. This state of play can often snowball and mutate, producing habits and beliefs that unfortunately become deep-rooted in people's minds. They are then translated into the next exercise philosophy, routine or regime.

Exercising and the relentless pursuit for the perfect module have succumbed to this process and many past and present protocols contain absolutely **no** scientific basis. The vast majority of exercise advice has come, and continues to come, from individuals who are simply **not qualified** to give such advice.

The exercise industry has, it seems, evolved into an industry where the accepted norm allows, even promotes, advice from self-proclaimed experts, social media stars, celebrities and exercise gurus.

PERSONAL BACKGROUND

With all their diversity and substantial volume, the 100,000 one-to-one personal training sessions that I have conducted have enabled me to judge, analyse and conclude countless common themes and patterns of response to exercise that I simply could not ignore. Scientific, psychological, medical and mechanical understanding of the human body have all developed immeasurably over my 37 years' experience.

Exercise is about using and enhancing the whole body's natural, organic, fluid, rhythmical movement patterns, allowing and achieving efficiency, symmetry, proportion and muscle, bone, and joint stability.

But despite all these advances, **THE WHOLE WORLD IS GETTING IT WRONG. YES, THE WHOLE WORLD IS GETTING IT WRONG.**

We've established that there really aren't any exercise specialists who specialise in *you*. In 2023, in my opinion, this is simply unacceptable. **You** have been forgotten, *you* have been confused and *you* have even been misled.

How do you choose whether to run or cycle, row, or use the stepper, lift heavy or lift light, do Pilates or yoga or boxing, or take part in classes? Can you be sure that you are choosing the right regime for *you*? Are you progressing or are you missing out on many elements that could be vital for your body, health and fitness?

In summary, despite the exercise and fitness boom of the last 35 to 40 years and the concurrent explosion in the number of personal trainers, the scientific understanding of human movement patterns is still neither being taught nor understood by the exercising masses.

To this day I come across people, clients, so-called professionals and even personal trainers who have absolutely no understanding of an individual's unique movement patterns and their vital importance, or of the compensatory forces that ravage the human skeleton, muscles and joints. They cannot therefore understand the critical need for exercise programmes that address these issues and are bespoke to each and every individual.

The last 40 years haven't seen any change in this state of affairs. We are still blinkered, still searching for the next miraculous must-try, one-size-fits-all regime. This simply must change, and must change now. The understanding of human movement has to be addressed and new methods, ideas and regimes have to be developed using scientific knowledge.

This is why I have always operated differently and why I have felt an enormous sense of duty to release my 'secret' philosophies, my ideas, my methods and hence my 100,000 exercise programmes.

Let my knowledge and experience educate and guide **you** to a better way to train that achieves better, faster results and longevity of movement and performance. And let's start by examining some of the fundamental myths, misconceptions and missing links that are holding you back.

Myths and Misconceptions

The unregulated fitness industry has **complicated, confused and even misled** every one of us. The relentless pursuit of the one-system-fits-all approach of the last 40 years has served only to produce so much conflicting information and advice that most individuals don't know which way to turn when deciding on exercise, and even the most basic of principles is misinterpreted or misunderstood. This has led to an ever-growing number of myths and misconceptions existing in the exercise world, muddying the waters, preventing scientific progress and holding us back.

Here are 40 of the most common.

1. *Exercising the abdominal muscles reduces belly fat*. This is absolute nonsense, of course.

Muscle and fat are completely different entities. Exercising a particular muscle or muscle group has absolutely no correlation with 'burning the fat away' in the same area. This applies to the abdominal area of the body and every other one.

Remember this analogy: starting with a full tank of fuel in your car, you can't ensure that you only burn the fuel from the middle part of the tank. It will simply deplete the more frequently, the faster and the longer you drive. So with the human body, your fat stores (fuel), will deplete gradually, slowly and uniformly, in direct relation to the frequency, intensity and duration of your exercising.

You simply can't 'spot-reduce' fat.

2. *Running is bad for your knees.* This is not true.

One of the key characteristics of the human being is that we are bipeds, having evolved to stand, walk and run on two legs. It is a fundamental part of our existence.

"Numerous studies have shown that runners have lower rates of knee osteoarthritis than sedentary people," according to runnersworld.com. Why, then, do so many people believe this myth? The answer is very simple but still misunderstood.

In Chapter 7 I will explain the complexities and importance of human biomechanics – the way we stand, walk and run. Technique, posture, foot contact, knee angles, hip/pelvis position and spinal position all dictate the mechanics of how we all move. This is a very personal chain reaction of movement, and unfortunately most individuals have less than perfect mechanics that can, and often do, put undue stress through the knee joint.

So an individual's poor biomechanics can be bad for their knees, but running doesn't have a direct effect. With good biomechanics, running can have very important benefits for an individual's knee muscles and joints.

This is one of the fundamental reasons why I have formulated my 100,000 system – I want to increase knowledge and understanding of the importance of mechanics and how to address them throughout the entire body.

3. *Exercise turns fat into muscle.* Not true.

As I've already stated, fat and muscle are completely different tissues and one cannot morph into another. Exercise can only decrease one (fat) and increase another (muscle).

4. *Core stability is everything.* This modern-day mantra is not true.

Many individuals don't fully understand what core stability is, what it does or how to exercise it correctly. Devoting too much time to simply exercising the abdominal area in a one-dimensional manner simply doesn't address the issue. It requires a multifaceted approach which, when executed correctly, is a very important component of exercise but no more important than many others.

Again, I have built my 100,000 system to include all the vital components that the human body requires to function fluidly and efficiently.

5. *No pain, no gain.* How many of us continually hear this untruth?

'Pain' is not the correct word to associate with anything that relates to exercise.

That said, to induce the exercise adaptations you're striving for, you must exercise frequently, intensely and with enough variety to encourage your body outside its comfort zone. Exercising to the required fatigue levels ensures that, during the body's rest periods, it recovers and super-compensates for the exercise that has been done. This is simply how the body works and progresses.

MYTHS AND MISCONCEPTIONS

6. *Workouts should always be one hour long.* Again, simply not true.

Exercise response is about consistent quality, not solely about quantity and volume. Remember one of my top tips – stretching your hamstrings for 60 seconds each, and/or 30 seconds of back mobility every day, could potentially cure the world of back pain.

7. *You can outrun a bad diet.* This is not strictly true.

If you're young and naturally slim or lean, with a fast metabolism, huge quantities of exercise can *appear* to be achieving the desired results, but don't be blindsided.

Please be aware that bad, unhealthy, fatty junk-food diets will destroy your health and build up fat somewhere in your body – for example in the form of deep fat around your vital organs – even if it's not being stored where it would be more visible, just under your skin.

8. *Sweating equals results.* Again, this needs clarification.

Some exercising may make us sweat, some may not, and we all sweat at different rates and to a different degree.

The scientific truth, is that, relative to your starting levels, you will sweat sooner after starting exercise, and you will sweat more, when you exercise continually/regularly for weeks or months. So monitoring your sweat rates can be a good indication of your progress.

9. *Stretching before exercise is crucial.* Similarly, this needs clarification.

The benefit depends on the type of stretching, what you're stretching, why you're stretching and how you're stretching. It also depends on what exercise is to follow.

Let's be clear: stretching, both statically and dynamically, is very important to the human body and important for muscles, nerves and the entire skeleton. Stretching performed correctly, at the correct times and in the correct balance, can and will be highly beneficial to your body.

10. *Lifting weights makes women bulk up.* Unless this is an individual's objective for their exercise, it's not generally correct.

Building muscle takes highly targeted exercise over an extended period – months or years – and therefore it's almost impossible to attain too much musculature without recognising it. It is also important to emphasise here how quickly (three or four days) muscles can atrophy (diminish in size), so scaling down muscular exercises can very quickly rectify any overdevelopment that may happen.

11. *Rowing is good for the stomach.* **This is a commonly held belief that makes no sense at all.**

The musculature in the stomach/abdominal area should be engaged during the rowing movement, but this applies to numerous other exercises, movements and activities and is not specific to the rowing action.

Good use of rowing exercise, as part of a comprehensive, varied and balanced cardiovascular exercise routine, is of course beneficial to the body's overall fat consumption, but not directly from the stomach region.

12. *To build your body, you have to use weights.* **Except in the case of advanced bodybuilding, this simply isn't correct.**

'Building' your body requires quality, variety and consistency of controlled muscular fatigue, and there are many other options other than weights that can achieve this.

13. *Sweating means you're not fit.* **This needs to be defined correctly.**

Sweating is the body's mechanism for regulating internal temperature. If your internal (core) temperature rises too high, the body diverts water to the skin surface to evaporate the heat out. An unfit, unhealthy and/or overweight individual may sweat simply as a response to having too much insulation in the form of fat, but the opposite may be true.

As one gets fitter, the body's thermoregulatory system becomes more efficient, recognising any heat build-up more quickly and acting quickly to remove it – sweating more, and sooner, to regulate body temperature. Indeed, individuals from opposite sides of the health/fitness spectrum both sweat profusely, but for completely opposing reasons.

14. *Stretching prevents injury.* **It really isn't as simple as this.**

As I've said, stretching generally is highly beneficial to the human body, especially as a tool to aid injury prevention, but it must be done correctly, be well balanced and

MYTHS AND MISCONCEPTIONS

be highly targeted to individuals. It certainly does not come with any guarantee.

15. *Cardiovascular exercise should always come first.* This simply isn't true.

Every exercising individual needs good quality, progressive cardiovascular exercise, and traditional gym exercise programmes usually schedule the cardiovascular component at the start of every workout.

However, my 100,000 exercise system has variety at its heart, especially because the best results are gained with a variety of movements and exercises and continued variety of routines. There is no definitive scientific evidence that cardiovascular exercise must come first.

16. *You should go to the gym daily.* Once again, this simply isn't accurate.

Doing any amount of exercise daily isn't recommended. It should also be remembered that even regular gym-goers do not always have to go to the gym to carry out effective exercise sessions. Over-training is in fact one of the most common problems for regular exercisers.

It must be remembered that, to progress, the body needs rest from exercise. In fact many adaptations from exercise come during the body's rest periods and not during the workout itself.

17. *You should never work out with an empty stomach.* This is false.

Good health and fitness depend on good nutrition, and that covers what you eat, how much you eat and when you eat. Elite athletes experiment extensively in order to establish what, how much and when to eat before training.

Scientifically speaking, exercising with a full stomach isn't clever. The human body requires a significant amount of blood and energy to digest food efficiently. If there is a physiological competition for blood supply between your digestive system and your exercising muscles, your muscles will win out every time.

That may sound good for your exercise, but it's a disaster for your digestive system. If it were a choice between full or empty, then empty should be the choice.

18. *Yoga isn't a proper workout.* This is untrue.

I believe that an individual shouldn't just practise yoga or only practise yoga, and there are some scientifically contraindicated (controversial) movements and positions in yoga, but there are also some highly effective and beneficial movements and positions. Every individual should include them in their workouts.

19. *Pilates isn't a proper workout.* **This again is completely incorrect.**

Pilates is currently in vogue, and although it clearly isn't the total answer to everyone's exercise needs, there are many important Pilates exercises that we should all incorporate into our workouts.

20. *Exercise is dangerous.* **This is a sweeping statement that is obviously incorrect.**

In reality, injury does happen during gym exercise but it's far less common than most people realise.

However, this does not change the fact that all exercise should be performed slowly, correctly and in a well thought-out, considered manner. This not only ensures that exercising is safe, it also ensures it is efficient and effective.

21. *Early morning is the best time to exercise.* **This is untrue.**

There are genetic factors that may determine an individual's favoured exercise time of day for exercise, but it hasn't been proved that, even for these individuals, it produces better results.

22. *Sports drinks are good.* **Unfortunately this isn't accurate.**

Most of them are complete junk.

23. *All exercisers need more protein.* **This is a very modern mantra.**

While it's true that serious exercisers may benefit from slightly more protein, it is simply not correct to guzzle protein drinks at every opportunity.

24. *Gaining weight means gaining fat.* **Another claim that is completely untrue.**

It is quite possible, even common, to lose fat and gain weight. This, of course, must mean that muscle tissue has been gained. Muscle tissue is denser (heavier) than fat and therefore a small increase in muscle mass can outweigh a reduction in body fat.

MYTHS AND MISCONCEPTIONS

25. *Sitting is the new smoking*. This statement, if taken literally, isn't true.

But recent scientific research has certainly highlighted the notion that a sedentary life is seriously bad for one's health.

'Never sit still for more than one hour at any one time' has become a mantra in some quarters. From a pure health perspective, constant activity is just as important as actual exercise, so the maxim does have some credibility.

26. *We should be less active as we age*. This is comprehensively untrue.

In fact, the opposite may be true; it depends on the exact definition of active. We certainly may need to modify our exercise choices and routines as we age, but in general we need to exercise more to stay the same, let alone continue to progress, as we age.

27. *You can't lose weight walking*. This is generally untrue; however, some clarification is needed.

Walking for an elite athlete, even over long distances, probably wouldn't produce any significant benefit (and they probably wouldn't be overweight), but walking can provide ideal weight loss conditions for many individuals. Much will depend on the intensity, speed and gradients.

28. *You burn more fat by exercising longer*. This is not strictly true.

The rate of burning fat is determined by a multitude of factors – intensity, duration, heart rate, breathing rate, frequency of exercise and metabolic rate, all of which need to be precise. On the other hand, you won't see too many overweight marathon runners.

29. *You need to be sore to progress*. This again is not strictly true.

It really depends on the definition of sore. Progression with muscular exercise does require muscular fatigue, and this does often go hand in hand with a certain degree of stiffness or slight soreness, but it's not a prerequisite for progress.

30. *Bigger muscles mean greater strength*. This is another one that is not strictly true.

Exercising for strength and exercising for size are not necessarily the same, and it's quite possible to be strong without being big. However, there is a degree of overlap, and in general, bigger muscles are stronger than smaller muscles.

31. *Running outdoors is better than running on a treadmill.* **This is not specifically true.**

There are small mechanical and impact differences between the two activities, but they're essentially the same.

32. *You have to do 20 minutes of cardio.* **No, it's not that simple.**

The established standard 30 years ago was that, for health and fitness benefits, everyone should strive for three cardiovascular sessions of 20 minutes every week. But recent scientific research has directed us towards greater regularity of exercise, combined with greater intensity.

It's important here to emphasise the importance of variety, and this includes variety of cardiovascular exercise. The regular gym-goer should vary their cardio workouts to include longer (up to one hour), medium-intensity sessions and shorter, sharper (30 seconds to five minutes) high-intensity bouts of cardio.

33. *Exercise machines are better than dumb-bells.* **This is not true.**

Some individuals do have preferences but there is a place for both in any gym exercise routine, and please remember the importance of variety.

34. *Working out makes you hungry.* **This is not strictly true.**

In the short term, an intense, prolonged bout of exercise may appear to stimulate hunger, but this is not an ongoing issue for exercisers. Remember that a healthy human body should develop hunger, but develop it to the correct level and at the right times.

35. *Treadmills are better than bikes, rowers and steppers.* **Essentially this isn't true.**

Your body doesn't know whether you're exercising on a treadmill, bike, rower or stepper – it only knows how hard it needs to work to supply the demands of the exercise through its heart rate, breathing rate, blood flow, energy consumption and so on. So the different forms of exercise are essentially the same.

MYTHS AND MISCONCEPTIONS

They entail, of course, different movements and therefore have different muscular involvement. Detailed analysis shows slight differences in these activities, and individuals differ in how they perceive their relative difficulties. Again, please remind yourself of the importance of variety in any workout.

36. *Lifting weights doesn't help weight loss.* This is untrue.

Weight loss is the result, the side effect, of exercising properly – correctly, consistently and effectively – and weight training is certainly a vital element of exercising properly.

37. *You must work out daily.* This is not necessary; indeed, it's imperative to give the body sufficient rest to facilitate the body's progression.

That said, there is only benefit to be gained from doing two to five minutes of some kind of activity during your rest days. This could be two minutes of spinal mobility or five minutes of stretching, especially if you have issues such as tightness or injuries to overcome.

38. *Lean muscle is different from bulk.* This is true.

The term 'bulk' usually refers to limb dimensions that encompass muscles, bones, fat, and skin – in other words, the total dimension. 'Lean muscle' refers solely to muscle dimensions.

39. *To be big, you must lift big.* This is not true.

Building or growing muscles requires a varied approach to muscular fatigue, which should incorporate light, medium and heavy weights.

For maximum muscle growth, however, there must be a high percentage contribution from a variety of 'heavy' weight exercises.

40. *We evolved to be physically active.* This is true.

And it's exactly why recent scientific research points us towards more general, regular, daily or even hourly activity.

All of these myths and misconceptions have served to misrepresent exercise, to cloud opinion and understanding. They have led to exercise becoming a guessing game with individuals simply following others, not really knowing if they are doing things correctly. It has been a major contributing factor to explain why exercise has been, and still is, so confusing to so many.

With all that said, there is one factor that remains elusive – a factor that has been completely overlooked and that is essential to each and every one of us. It's a **fundamental missing link** that should, **must** underpin every exercise programme, routine or regime.

As a sport scientist, I have always seen and done things differently. I have always respected the fact that the 'personal' in personal trainer is not about me, it's about my client – it's about **you**. As a sport scientist, I appreciate that understanding the way **you** sit, stand, walk and move is imperative if I am to come to an understanding of **you**. Without this understanding, prescribing bespoke exercise programmes becomes a guessing game, with your results being in the lap of the gods.

But what is this missing link? What are these movement patterns? The study and science of human movement is called HUMAN BIOMECHANICS. Let's have a closer look at this important science and explain why it's such a crucial missing link.

The **missing link** – human **biomechanics**

The fundamental factor that should and must underpin your exercise programme is **you**.

That means **your** body, **your** proportions and strengths, **your** weaknesses and imbalances, **your** flexibility, **your** muscles and joints, **your** posture, **your** range of movement, **your** feet, legs, hips, and pelvis, **your** back, **your** neck, shoulders and arms, **your** body type, **your** stance, **your** movement and **your** physiological make-up. It is everything that makes you unique.

But what is it about you that makes you a unique individual?

We are an extremely complex array of muscles, ligaments, tendons, nerves, bones, joints and segments that must all perform as a well-oiled machine, reacting consistently and fluidly with millisecond timing in order for us to move, walk, run, sit, stand, jump, lift, carry, twist and bend efficiently.

One thing is often misunderstood or even completely overlooked: the understanding that the movement of one segment (for example the knee) has consequences for the next segment (for example the hips and pelvis) and the next (the spine) and so on, throughout the entire body from head to toe. This sequence or chain reaction is known as the human kinetic chain and the scientific understanding of this complex sequence is known as **human biomechanics** – the *mechanics of human movement*.

Even though most of us have two feet, two legs, two hips, a pelvis, a spine and two arms, and generally move in a similar way, we all have a unique and personal movement pattern sequence. At first glance this sequence appears universal, but with detailed scrutiny significant imperfections may, and usually do, appear. The knowledge, the understanding of these imperfections is critical. Understanding how, and more importantly **why you** move the way you do is vital in compiling **your** exercise programmes. We all need a much greater understanding of our own **unique kinetic chain of movement**.

THE MISSING LINK – HUMAN BIOMECHANICS

A full scientific, mathematical biomechanical analysis of the human body while running, jumping, twisting, bending, reaching, catching, throwing, swimming, rowing, squatting or lunging – not to mention swinging a golf club, hitting a tennis serve or kicking a football – is eye-watering in its complexity.

Even when something as simple as walking (gait) is given a full biomechanical analysis, it becomes abundantly clear that perfect or near-perfect movement patterns are nothing short of miraculous.

First, let's consider our feet. The foot, which gives us the ability to walk upright, is unique to humans. It has developed specifically to adapt to the surface on which we walk.

In the early stages of our evolution the Earth's terrain was varied and uneven, and the foot has a complex set of joints and muscles that allow this process. However, we are now required to walk on hard, flat, man-made surfaces, subjecting the foot and legs to low-grade but repetitive movement.

For most of us, simply putting one foot in front of the other and walking is something that we take for granted; we never give it a second thought. So let's consider a simplified biomechanical breakdown of the forces, muscles, bones and joints and the movements that take place during one stride (one gait cycle). This is from when a heel strikes the ground until the same heel contacts the ground for a second time.

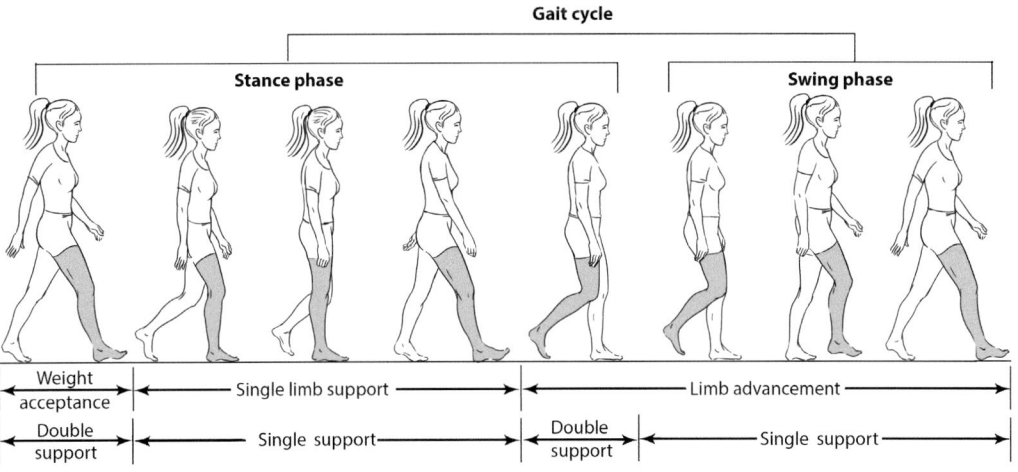

THE MISSING LINK – HUMAN BIOMECHANICS

The requirements of the body during each gait cycle are as follows:

1. **Weight acceptance**
2. **Single leg support**
3. **Limb advancement**

The gait cycle itself is categorised in two phases.

1. **The stance phase** – this phase encompasses 60 to 62 per cent of the cycle. This phase alone is broken down into five biomechanical stages as follows:

   a. Initial contact (heel strike) – two per cent
      – Double support
   b. Loading response – ten per cent
      – Contralateral toe off
   c. Mid stance – 19 per cent
   d. Terminal stance – 19 per cent
      – Contralateral stance
   e. Pre-swing – 12 per cent

2. **The swing phase.** This phase consists of 38 to 40 per cent of the total gait cycle and is made up of three stages as follows:

   a) Initial swing (toe off) – 13 per cent
   b) Mid swing – 12 per cent
   c) Terminal swing – 13 per cent

During the analysis of this gait cycle, it is imperative to assess the following positions and movements:

a. Hip/pelvic alignment, which we usually refer to as hip drop, on either or both sides.
b. Hiking – excess lifting of segments on either or both sides.
c. Backward/forward lean – excess leaning forwards (flexion) or backwards (extension).
d. Excess rotations – excess twisting/rotation of hips, pelvis, spine and shoulders. To assess these angles and movements accurately, we must analyse the gait cycle from different angles.
1. The side view (sagittal plane). From this view we can clearly assess the bending (flexion) and straightening (extension) for the ankle, knee and hips, checking for the angle of the pelvis (pelvic tilt) and curvature of the lower

back (lumbar lordosis).
2. The front/back view (coronal plane). Here we must check for the collapsing in (adduction) or the bowing out (abduction) of the thigh bone (femur), knock knees (knee valgus), bowed knees (knee varus) and low/flat foot arches (pronation), high foot arches (supination) and pelvis position (pelvic obliquity).
3. The above view (transverse/axial plane). Here we are assessing trunk, leg and pelvis rotations and the foot progression angle.

Also, during the gait cycle there is a complex array of different highly coordinated muscle contractions, as follows:

1. Concentric muscle contractions. This is where the muscle is shortening under load.
2. Isometric muscle contractions, where the muscle maintains its length under load.
3. Eccentric muscle contractions. This is where the muscle is lengthening under load.

Analysing muscle activity in a little more detail reveals intricate millisecond timing, as follows:

The lower leg muscles:

a. The plantar flexors.
   The calf muscles (gastrocnemius and soleus).
   – Inactivity during the heel strike and loading response phase.
   – Eccentric contractions to control dorsiflexion during the mid-stance phase.
   – Concentric contractions to propel the body forwards during the heel and toe-off phase.
   – These muscles control rhythm, speed, timing and balance.
   Tibialis posterior, flexor hallucis longus, flexor digitorum longus.
   – Eccentric contractions during the loading response phase to control the degree of pronation.
b. The dorsiflexors (tibialis anterior, extensor digitorum longus, extensor hallucis longus).
   – Eccentric contractions during the heel strike phase to control plantar flexion, preventing foot 'slap'.
   – Isometric contractions during the swing phase.

The thigh muscles:

a. The quadriceps (rectus femoris, vastus lateralis, vastus intermedius, vastus medialis).
   – Eccentric contractions during heel strike to control knee flexion.
   – Concentric contractions during loading response phase for forward propulsion.
   – Inactivity during the mid-terminal stance phases.
   – Eccentric contractions during the heel and toe-off phases to control knee flexion.
   – Eccentric contractions during the swing phase.
b. The hamstrings (biceps femoris, semimembranosus, semitendinosus).
   – Eccentric contractions during heel strike phase to control flexion.
   – Concentric contractions during the loading response phase to extend the hip.
   – Eccentric contractions during the swing phase to control the speed of movement.

The hip/pelvis muscles:

a. The gluteus maximus.
   – Eccentric contraction during heel strike phase to resist flexion.
   – Concentric contraction during loading response phase to extend the hip.
   – Inactivity during the pre-swing phase.
   – Eccentric contraction during the swing phase to slow hip flexion.
b. The gluteus medius.
   – Eccentric contraction during heel strike phase to control the pelvis.
   – Concentric contraction as the knee extends to accept body weight and propel the body forward.
   – These muscles are crucial for stabilisation of the pelvis.
c. Adductor magnus.
   – Eccentric contraction during the toe-off phase to stabilise the pelvis.
d. Iliopsoas.
   – Eccentric contraction during the mid-stance phase to resist extension.
   – Concentric contraction during the swing phase to flex the hip.

The trunk muscles:

a. Erector spinae.
   – Eccentric contraction during heel strike phase to prevent forward bend.

During the gait cycle, as the leg accepts floor contact (ground reaction force) and weight, the force that the knee accepts/absorbs is equal to approximately two to three times total bodyweight. This represents highly significant forces that the body has to absorb, and please remember that these huge forces represent the mechanics of just one stride.

This is a simplified biomechanical analysis, but I'm sure you would agree that it shows the human body's movement patterns are highly complex and intricate. These patterns are a highly involved kinetic chain of actions and reactions that requires millisecond timing to produce the rhythmical movement of something as simple as walking, but it's vital to understand that these patterns are unique to each individual.

Whilst this gait movement relies on split-second timing, there is a range of acceptability of about five degrees of deviation for normal lift and rotation. Importantly, however, as an example, just between three and five degrees of deviation in tibial valgus (internal rotation) alignment of the lower leg can induce a 50 per cent increase in force transmitted across the medial (internal) tibio-femoral compartment of the knee.

Between three and five degrees of deviation is minuscule, but it's not too difficult to understand that a 50 per cent increase in force engulfing the knee joint can have serious consequences, not only for the knee but at **any** point up through the entire kinetic chain.

These consequences represent issues that each and every one of us should and must understand. This is where the human body starts to compensate. Slight deviations in foot, ankle or knee mechanics could produce compensatory patterns that over time ravage the musculoskeletal system, leading to niggles, aches, pains or injuries anywhere throughout the human body.

When the deviations of movement consistently fall significantly outside 'normal' gait ranges, there are well-known, well-established classifications for the resulting patterns of movement. There are in fact, apart from 'normal' gait, eight other pathological gait patterns that can be attributed to musculoskeletal neurological conditions, as follows:

1. Trendelenburg/myopathic gait. This, named after the surgeon Friedrich Trendelenburg, is an abnormal gait pattern resulting from a defective hip abduction mechanism, where there is weakness or ineffective action of the gluteus medius and gluteus minimus muscles.

2. Hemiplegic gait. This is an abnormal gait pattern where the leg is stiff, without flexion at the knee and ankle.

3. Diplegic gait is an abnormal gait pattern characterised by a narrow base and dragging both legs and scraping the toes.

4. Neuropathic gait. This is an abnormal gait pattern characterised by foot drop and/or ankle drop due to loss of dorsiflexion.

5. Choreiform gait is an abnormal gait pattern, presenting a mixed pattern of unpredictable accelerations and decelerations – twisting choreitic movements of the trunk, head, arms and legs.

6. Ataxic gait is an abnormal gait described as a staggering gait pattern.

7. Parkinson's gait. This is an abnormal gait pattern characterised by small shuffling steps.

8. Sensory gait is an abnormal gait classified by a lack of coordination.

All of these gait patterns need very careful attention as they put very significant demands on the human body. Although they are very real, they are quite rare, but even 'normal' gait can stray towards these extreme patterns with too much repetitive movement.

For example, consider the modern-day trend of the 10,000-steps-a-day regime. We have seen the complexity, the room for deviation, of just one stride and its associated forces, so just imagine the accumulative anatomical stress, the biomechanical consistency, needed to absorb this huge number of repeated kinetic chain reactions.

Furthermore, it's now clear to see that exercises like jogging or running must increase the potential for further deviations in our biomechanical functioning, reducing efficiency, especially when we realise that the impact forces during jogging or running multiply to approximately four times our total bodyweight. This represents a tremendously increased load that the skeleton has to endure, stride after stride after stride.

If you have perfect or near-perfect biomechanics your body can absorb and compensate for these extra forces beautifully, like a well-oiled machine, but as I have stated, because of its extreme complexity it would be nothing short of a **miracle** to have such perfect biomechanics. My own, slightly imperfect biomechanics as a 16-year-old was the root cause of a knee injury that might have put paid to a flourishing professional sporting career.

Over the years I have repeatedly seen this biomechanical pattern affecting client after client after client, from beginners to elite sportsmen and women, regardless of age, height, weight, body type, balance, posture and athleticism. It was affecting almost every one of my clients to some extent.

These biomechanical inefficiencies explain why so many individuals suffer niggles, aches, pains and injuries arising from many activities. **How are your biomechanics affecting you?** Have you ever even thought about how your feet, ankles, knees, hips and pelvis function?

What's more, I can conclude from years of experience that THE WORLD IS FULL OF BACK PAIN. A very high percentage of this is caused by inefficiency in one's biomechanics. In explanation, let me extrapolate further.

I have always compared our gluteal muscle group and pelvis to the foundations necessary when building a new house. Without these unseen foundations, even the most majestically designed and built house will eventually crumble and fall to the ground, preceded by many movement cracks as the house tries to remain upright.

Imagine, then, that our gluteal muscles are tight, weak or simply not functioning optimally, leading to a constantly collapsing motion of our pelvis from side to side as we walk, jog or run. Add to this even slight foot pronation (collapsing inwards) and we have the classic scenario of what we have already termed *hip drop* (Trendelenburg gait). This effectively results in a constant 'rocking' of the pelvis and therefore an unstable foundation for the spine to sit on. This is far more common than anyone ever seems to understand.

The ongoing consequence of this 'rocking' is **spinal compensation**. Repeated spinal compensations over a short term are absorbed beautifully by the human body, but in the mid to long term continued compensations lead to tight muscles and tight joints that become locked. This in turn leads to niggles, aches, pains and injuries. Sometimes these compensations lead to lifelong underlying, low-level pain that so many of us learn to live with.

This is simply not acceptable.

The human spine is an incredible structure. The 'normal' spine has 33 vertebrae that form an S-shaped curve when viewed from the side. This shape allows for an even distribution of weight and flexibility of movement. This normal-shaped spine can perform actions to marvel at – look at the astonishing movements and actions of a pole vaulter, high jumper or gymnast, for example.

Scoliosis, kyphosis and lordosis are the names given to the various curvatures of the human spine.

- Scoliosis is the side-to-side (lateral) curvature.
- Kyphosis is a forward curve that shifts the centre of balance in front of the hips.
- Lordosis is a concave lower back that thrusts the hips forward.

Mechanically, human movement affords a small (five to ten per cent) range of deviation from the normal ranges before there are any serious compensatory factors involved. Scoliosis, kyphosis and lordosis greater than the acceptable range of deviation can start to have very serious consequences reverberating through the entire length of the spine.

Exaggerated scoliosis, kyphosis and/or lordosis can occur from birth or develop from a whole host of reasons, ranging from growth abnormalities, postural habits, trauma, ageing and surgery to degeneration, disease or infection. One of the main factors, however, is constant repetitious movements with poor biomechanics.

This is something that I experience every day: the vast majority of my clients experience some degree of back pain. Poor biomechanics can negatively influence our muscles, bones and joints in an upward direction, from the feet up through the body, or in a downward direction, from the head and neck down through the body.

On consideration of this highly detailed sequencing of human movement, it's clear that if only one link in the chain is slightly and consistently 'off perfect', the whole sequencing becomes flawed, imperfect and inefficient, which inevitably has significant consequences on the body. But there are unfortunately many other factors that queue up to test the efficiency of this human chain reaction:

- A dominant side. Most of us are born right– or left-handed. This inevitably leads to favouring the dominant side, which in turn leads to unequal forces through the human kinetic chain.
- Body weight. Being overweight or underweight can lead to extra stresses through the musculoskeletal system.

- Postural habits or issues. Good posture is vital for fluent gait movement, but very few individuals have and maintain good posture, especially during intense exercising and sporting movements.
- Limb dimensions. It should not be assumed that all individuals have identical limb dimensions, with symmetry from side to side. Asymmetry imparts a great stress through the human body's kinetic chain.
- Activities/habits. Habits, by definition, evolve from continued repeated positions and movements. Non-symmetrical positions and movements can lead to asymmetrical mechanics.
- Tight muscles. Overly tight muscles restrict joints, affecting the fluidity of human movement.
- Medical history. Many medical conditions can have adverse effects on the human body's movement patterns.
- Age. Ageing can influence limb range of movement and flexibility, and hence human mechanics.
- Over-training certain elements. Over-training generally, and specifically the over-training of repetitious single dimension movements, can compromise the musculoskeletal system.
- Leg length discrepancy (LLD) is a major factor affecting gait patterns. This is discussed in more detail in the next chapter.

Leg length discrepancy (LLD)

All of the additional factors outlined above only serve to further explain why perfect gait patterns are almost impossible to achieve consistently. Let's consider just one of these additional factors.

Imagine that your dining table had legs of different length. Obviously, your table would be wholly unstable, moving and rocking, with everything resting on it sliding and moving around. Similarly, if the human body has one leg longer than the other, any degree of efficiency or stability in the chain reaction sequence detailed above becomes impossible to achieve. It becomes completely apparent that significant consequences would arise if a leg length discrepancy existed.

If such a discrepancy were a particularly rare occurrence, of course it wouldn't be a dominant factor in human movement. It has, however, been said, researched many times and generally understood that up to 90 to 95 per cent of humans have a leg length discrepancy of some degree.

There is a belief that an acceptable range of variation/discrepancy of up to 1.1 centimetres exists. My experience has shown that discrepancies greater than this exist in abundance, and more importantly, even small (less than 1.1cm) discrepancies lead to some form of compensatory patterns that cause the vast majority of people to suffer. These discrepancies can significantly affect knee, hip, sacroiliac and pelvic mechanics.

For fluid, efficient human movement patterns, a symmetrical, well-aligned musculoskeletal system is essential. With symmetrical biomechanical movement, the human body can move and function with seemingly computerised rhythm, timing, speed, balance and fluidity, like a well-oiled machine. The reverse, of course, is also true – bad alignment and bad symmetry induce a multitude of compensatory reactions that can significantly reduce the efficiency of movement, increasing stress and fatigue throughout the entire human kinetic chain.

Symmetry of movement, therefore, is vitally important for sports and exercise. Unfortunately, almost none of us are structurally or fundamentally symmetrical – in essence, **we are all flawed**.

LEG LENGTH DISCREPANCY (LLD)

While the human body can be majestic in its capability to compensate adequately for asymmetry, when LLD is minimal, it must be remembered that this is very much an individual response, as even the most negligible discrepancies can be exposed during highly repetitive movements like jogging or running.

Logically, larger LLD puts greater stress through our muscles, bones and joints and induce much greater compensatory patterns. Put simply, repeated movements with such discrepancies can fundamentally change our biomechanics – our default movement patterns become out of kilter.

Even though the occurrence of LLD is so widespread, it should never be accepted as the norm, overlooked or dismissed. It's imperative that *you* understand *your* leg length function, and understand how it might be affecting *you*. Is it the cause of *your* knee, hip or back pain?

There are three types of leg length discrepancy:

1. **Structural.**
2. **Functional.**
3. **Environmental.**

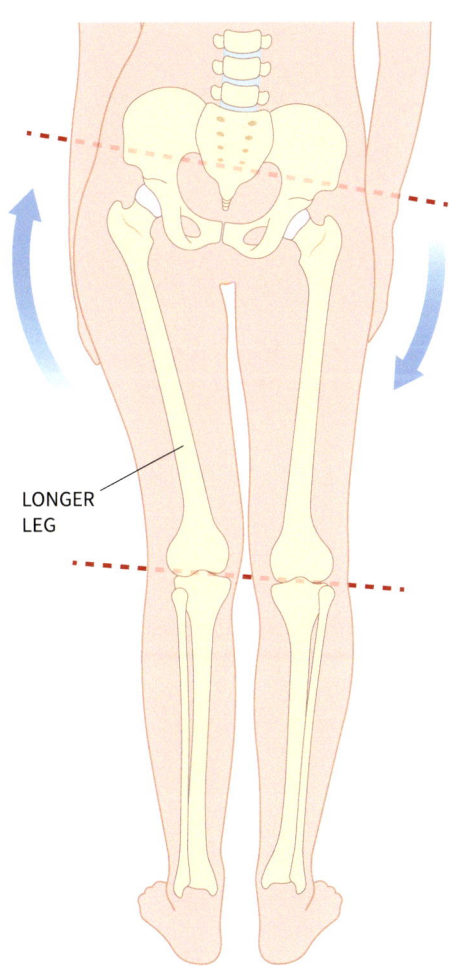

The structural or anatomical type is due to a difference in the actual length of the bones, usually the tibia (lower leg bone) or femur (thigh bone). This may be congenital, due to injuries or accidents, fractures, trauma or degenerative disease, or occur after surgery.

The functional type is due to asymmetry of the human biomechanical chain reaction of movement. This can occur at any point through this chain, from foot pronation or supination, knee valgum or varum, asymmetric hip function, spinal curvatures, resulting from muscle tightness, injuries and/or postural habits.

LEG LENGTH DISCREPANCY (LLD)

Differentiation of these two types of leg length difference is not always straightforward since it is not unusual to have both occur together.

The environmental type is caused by incorrect footwear, asymmetrical shoe wear or walking, jogging or running on different surfaces. This third type may exist independently or be an additional pathologic influence to an existing functional and/or structural leg length discrepancy.

If you reflect on the above information, it becomes abundantly clear that leg length discrepancies alone can be wholly destructive to an otherwise symmetrical biomechanical flow of movement.

"Where leg length discrepancies are over an acceptable range of difference, passive structural changes give way to active muscular compensatory movements." (Physiopedia)

I believe we can all understand and agree on this, but what is the acceptable range of difference? As mentioned above, the average LLD is less than 1.1 centimetres. However, as we have found, human biomechanics is highly individual in its sequencing and many studies conclude varying degrees of acceptability – even as much as 30 to 40 millimetres in some cases.

With my experience of working with thousands of different unique individuals, I can conclude with a very high degree of confidence that it doesn't always correlate that those with the greatest discrepancies suffer the most. While it's a logical assumption that greater discrepancies cause greater problems, I can report that some individuals with discrepancies greater than 1 to 1.5 inches do not seem to suffer any tangible adverse mechanical affects, while the converse is also true – some individuals who present LLD of only one to two millimetres can present significant musculoskeletal consequences.

This seemingly random response does not recommend itself to exercise programme prescription, but in my opinion – and indeed, in my experience – this should be seen as a truly positive situation, as it makes it even more imperative that we see ourselves and others as unique in our individual requirements from exercise.

Putting this simply, it is imperative that we all check for leg length discrepancies at the outset of initiating any exercise programme. It's important to realise here that the accurate, in-depth, medical procedure for measurement of leg length is

LEG LENGTH DISCREPANCY (LLD)

quite complex. It involves radiography and/or computed tomography (CT scan). Both procedures must be performed by specialists and can prove costly.

For the last 37 years I have employed a much more direct approach to judgement of leg length discrepancies. This method is so quick, easy and simple that it can be used by everyone.

This simple test is a **golden rule** to which you must adhere. This is the starting point; the establishing of any leg length discrepancy is the first part of understanding **your** biomechanics and the first indication of what makes **you, you**.

For this test, you will need a partner.

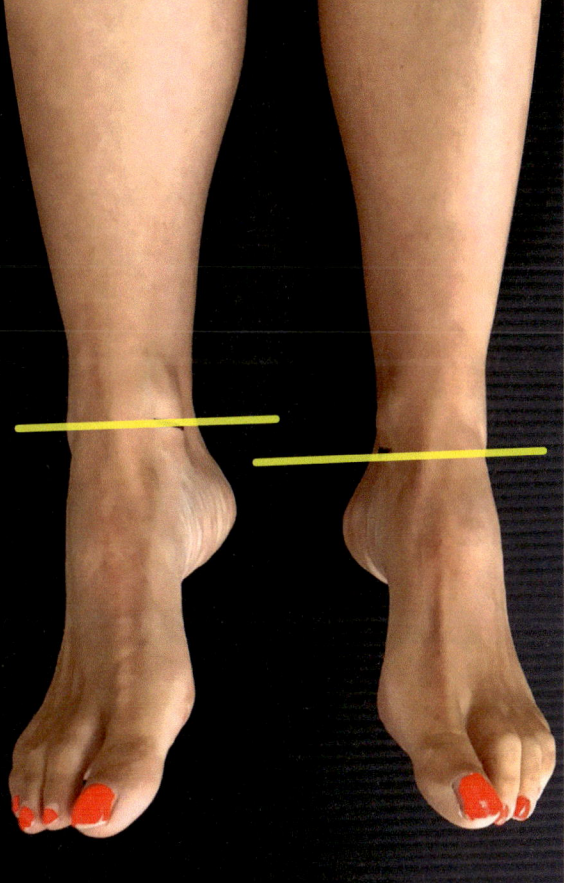

- Simply lie down flat on your back on the floor (a firm surface).
- Bend both knees, keep your feet on the ground and raise your hips off the ground, then slowly lower your hips back to the ground and straighten your legs (this puts you in the 'neutral' position).
- Get your partner to place his or her thumbs just under (at the base of) your right and left ankle bones (medial malleolus).
- Visual judgement of any discrepancy in thumb position will indicate any leg length discrepancy.
- This can also be done by marking (with a black marker pen) the same right and left ankle bone positions – see right.

LEG LENGTH DISCREPANCY (LLD)

This process literally takes ten seconds and, although it cannot be millimetre accurate, it is more than adequate to discover if any significant leg length discrepancy exists. If it does, then it must be taken seriously. The potential for you to display inefficient biomechanics is significant and must be addressed. My 100,000 exercise system is designed for you, to account for such discrepancies.

Any discrepancies discovered using this very simple test, however, do not clarify whether you have a structural and/or a functional and/or an environmental leg length discrepancy. Minor discrepancies, and more obviously, major discrepancies that are also accompanied by significant symptoms (foot, ankle, knee, hip or back pain) ideally need further exploration.

My 100,000 exercise system is ideal for such discrepancies, but establishing a 'true' structural leg length discrepancy is vital for long-term health and not just for shorter-term exercise choices. Indeed, even if there aren't any current symptoms, any significant discrepancies should ideally be examined further.

I have encountered all of these various scenarios on thousands of occasions. This is why I have put so much emphasis on such structural/stability issues and incorporated all the necessary exercises into my 100,000 routines. When I'm faced with such leg length discrepancies, using my experience, I analyse the functioning of the hips and pelvis and specifically the sacroiliac joint (where the lower spine meets the pelvis).

It's crucial but it doesn't occur in the normal training and education of most personal trainers, teachers and coaches. This is also in desperate need of change as the incidence of sacroiliac joint problems is prolific, especially in individuals who present leg length discrepancies. Personalised exercise programmes simply cannot be designed accurately without the knowledge and testing of leg length and sacroiliac function. Sacroiliac stability exercises also constitute an important part of my 100,000 system.

Consider then the enormous extra stress put on this highly tested, complex, uniquely human biomechanical chain if an individual presents a leg length discrepancy and any of the aforementioned factors – foot pronation, hip drop, knee valgum, bad posture, being overweight or scoliosis and so on – while sprinting, long-distance running, explosive jumping, in dynamic rotational movements in golf, tennis, gymnastics, athletics, cricket or baseball, changes in direction in team sports, squatting, lunging, weight training, high-intensity training and all other gym work.

LEG LENGTH DISCREPANCY (LLD)

Any combination of the above needs to be fully investigated if we are to be able to fully understand the intricate nature and combination of exercises necessary for you to manage your weaknesses and flourish with your exercising. This is where my 100,00 exercise system is so comprehensive and unique.

In summary, it is clear to see from the above that human biomechanics is highly complex. From detailed foot contact, a highly sequenced movement pattern moves up through the ankles, knees, hips, spine, neck and shoulders with majestic, sublime coordination and timing. However, its sheer complexity dictates that even if one link in the chain deviates from perfect, the whole chain becomes inefficient and the inevitable consequence and everyday reality is that it's practically impossible for the body to have the necessary posture, balance and symmetry needed to prevent a host of compensatory reactions throughout the entire human kinetic chain of movement.

It may at first sight be difficult to believe that such a delicate, fragile situation exists – especially during the exercise boom, when we are all exercising regularly, going to the gym regularly and have various regimes to choose from. Surely we should all be fitter, stronger, healthier, more subtle and flexible and hence in better physical condition. The following statistics, however, suggest a different picture.

World Health Organisation data (2019) showed that approximately 1.71 billion people globally live with musculoskeletal conditions, with lower back pain being the major contributor with more than 600 million prevalent cases in 2020. That number looks set to rise to nearly 850 million by 2050.

The Global Orthopaedic Surgery report 2017-2022 states: "In 2017, the number of orthopaedic surgery procedures performed worldwide totalled approximately 22.3 million. The number of procedures per year is forecast to grow at a 4.9 per cent compound annual rate over the 2017-2022 interval, approaching 28.3 million by 2022 and making this one of the most rapidly growing surgical procedure categories." The primary types of orthopaedic surgeries are hip and knee replacements. In 2013 / 2014 in England alone, there were 1.2 million orthopaedic procedures, with 115,758 hip replacements and 81,590 knee replacements.

In the UK there are more than 2,500 general surgeons and, more specifically, more than 2,000 orthopaedic surgeons dealing with various musculoskeletal operations, of which there are approximately:

1. 2,900 ankle procedures per annum, consisting of 2,000 arthrodesis and 900 full ankle replacements.

LEG LENGTH DISCREPANCY (LLD)

2. 21,000 shoulder operations a year in the UK and 1.4 million per annum globally.

3. More than 250,000 spinal procedures in 2017/2018, consisting of 211,000 pain relief injections and more than 52,500 surgical interventions.

It has been reported that all types of back pain cost the NHS more than £5 billion every year – an astronomical, almost unbelievable figure. Approximately eight million UK adults report chronic back pain every year, and back pain alone accounts for 40 per cent of workplace sickness – it's the number one reason for all long-term workplace sickness.

The cost of this to the UK economy is estimated at between £10 billion and £20 billion every year, and in the United States the annual cost is between $100 billion and $200 billion. This is one major reason why the British Orthopaedic Society concludes that there is a "growing musculoskeletal disease burden".

No wonder the World Health Organisation launched the Rehabilitation 2030 initiative in 2017 to draw attention to the "profound unmet need for rehabilitation worldwide".

Skeletal compensation leads to injury

There is no denying the enormity of the statistics quoted in the last chapter, but let's not be deflected from the realisation that they are compiled from various tangible research sources – they all come from actual medical recorded data. So they only include the number of cases that have been presented to the medical system, from doctor to operating table.

The real sobering fact is the realisation that although 80 per cent of adults suffer from some back pain, only seven per cent of them actually go to their doctor. This implies that the reality of back pain is that the vast majority of sufferers just try to or learn to live with the pain.

This is certainly backed up by my own empirical evidence concerning back pain from my 37 years' experience of working with thousands of people. By the time we encompass foot, ankle, knee, hip, shoulder and neck pain, we are unfortunately only then getting to the reality of the situation.

This proves to me that **everyone** is still getting it wrong. The exercise boom over the last 37 years is not resulting in better, fitter, stronger, more well-balanced human bodies. It is in fact having the opposite effect. The vast majority of regular exercisers are living with niggles, aches and pains of the feet, ankles, knees, hips, back, spine, neck and shoulders, and this has become the acceptable norm.

In my opinion, this simply cannot be acceptable and cannot continue. In fact, my knowledge and experience have proved that this does not need to be the consequence of the exercising generation. My 100,000 exercise system is designed to address and change this *'pandemic'*.

Let's consider the following scenario, an example of the status quo that still exists in 2023. How many of you can relate to having a sore knee from running, outdoors or on a treadmill in the gym? Initially you try to ignore it, convincing yourself that it will miraculously disappear. When inevitably it doesn't, you resort to painkillers. This often tempers the problem temporarily, although it rarely solves the problem.

You then decide to struggle on with your 30-minute sessions until the pain flares

SKELETAL COMPENSATION LEADS TO INJURY

up again. You then 'invest' in a miracle knee support bandage, again producing limited or no results. From there you try to cut back on your sessions to try to establish an acceptable volume of weekly running, which again produces some relief but is rarely satisfactory.

Unfortunately, at this point you might give up on your exercise altogether, or maybe learn to live with the daily low-level pain that you can just about tolerate as long as you don't do anything too strenuous. Only if this pain becomes unbearable do you then decide that you must go to visit your doctor. If your doctor is sympathetic, he or she might decide to send you for an x-ray or MRI scan. This scenario is all too familiar – and of course, it can relate to any part of the human body.

You might conclude from this example that I am going to recommend that you should all head off to your doctors at the onset of any slight discomfort. This is absolutely not the case – let me explain why.

Even if any discomfort or pain is minimal, a doctor or even a knee (orthopaedic) specialist will assume that knee pain emanates from the knee joint. This seems highly logical, but it is not always the case – most knee pain for a regular exerciser comes from biomechanical movement, and not from the knee joint specifically.

Let me be clear: x-rays and MRI scans are incredible advances in medical science but, clearly, they only observe the inside of a joint when it is stationary. It is then all too common to assume that any deterioration or wear and tear observed must correlate to the pain being experienced. This is simply not the case. This is where we all need a complete change of understanding and a change of approach.

As this, and many other examples stem from movement inefficiencies, it is surely obvious that we all need to analyse our movement patterns to understand why we may be suffering, or indeed have the potential to suffer, significant discomfort and/or pain. This leads me on to one of the key elements of my 100,000 system.

Movement analysis

We have seen from the alarming statistics above that, despite the boom in exercise participation and the plethora of fitness options, it is still abundantly clear that the current state of play is simply not working – as an exercising world, we are getting worse, not better.

You are not doing things correctly!

I have lived and worked with this issue, every hour of every day for the last 37 years, so this has become my driving force, my motivation for developing my 100,000 system and for writing this book.

How, though, do we rectify this? Do we need more doctors, more specialists, more x-rays, more MRI scans, more operations? **No!**

Quite clearly, I have shown that the vast majority of problems lie in an individual's movement patterns – their biomechanics. So movement – *your* movement – is exactly what we need to analyse.

This is the change, the shift and the education **everyone** needs. It provides the fundamental missing link that addresses and understands where and why everyone is going wrong.

This must now be the starting point, *your* education, for *you*. It will be an education in *your* stance, *your* posture, *your* foot and ankle movement, *your* knee position, *your* hip angles, *your* spinal position and curvature and *your* shoulder alignment.

If you can understand yourself, you can exercise more effectively and set your body free to move and function fluidly and efficiently and achieve your desired results more quickly. If you respect your skeleton, and look after it, it will look after you.

This is why I started as a personal trainer 37 years ago – I wanted to make your exercise about *you*. It is crucial for your understanding and hence your success, so use my knowledge and experience to learn about yourself. Over my career

MOVEMENT ANALYSIS

I have always analysed the human body from the inside out, starting with the skeleton and its movement.

I have explained that computing precise and scientifically accurate biomechanical data is highly complex, requiring highly trained scientists in a technically advanced laboratory, using very complex procedures and software, but let me show you how simple it can be for every one of you to get a real insight into your unique biomechanical movements. It really can be so easy, so quick and so simple that anyone can do it, and you need to do it now.

This is my **Golden Rule Number Four**.

To understand movement, we need to film movement. Thirty-seven years ago we didn't have a simple way of doing this, but these days almost all of us have mobile phones and can not only take video footage quickly and easily, but more importantly, use the slow-motion option that most mobile phones have.

Significant deviations in posture, stance, joint position and movement can be analysed easily with the naked eye, but slow-motion analysis is crucial for analysing the small nuances of an individual's movement patterns that are so commonplace, and so vital to understanding how you stand and move.

Instructions on how to self-analyse

- First, wear suitable attire – bare feet, shorts and a vest or T-shirt – to allow for good vision of all joints.
- Secondly, video-record four or five normal strides of the whole body from the front view.
- Thirdly, video-record four or five normal strides of the whole body from the rear view.
- Fourthly, video-record four or five normal strides of the whole body from a side view.
- Before replaying your video, take a picture of the stationary you.

The following is what you must look out for.

- Front view: good stance or posture is represented by clear horizontal alignment – specifically, ankles, knees, hips and shoulders.
- Side view: good stance or posture is represented with clear vertical alignment – specifically, head, shoulders, hips, knees and ankles.

MOVEMENT ANALYSIS

We rarely study our own stance or posture, so it's a subject to which we devote very little thought, importance or emphasis. We all stand so automatically that we really have no idea where our limbs, bones and joints lie in relation to good postural alignment. This was an issue that I uncovered very early in my career, and that's why I have always placed so much emphasis on the human skeleton. An unbalanced human frame, in a stationary stance, can have an enormous impact on your physical health.

Quite clearly, misalignment of your feet, ankles, knees, hips, spine and/or shoulders can lead to many niggles, aches, and pains of various kinds throughout your skeletal system, putting significant extra stress through your joints, musculature, ligaments and tendons. This misalignment can have serious consequences for the human body even when it's completely stationary. Imagine, therefore, the consequences of any kind of movement, exercise or sport on the musculoskeletal system.

The study of your movement patterns in slow motion, from different angles, is therefore crucial. The following diagrams represent a skeletal analogy of the adaptations that occur during something as simple as walking.

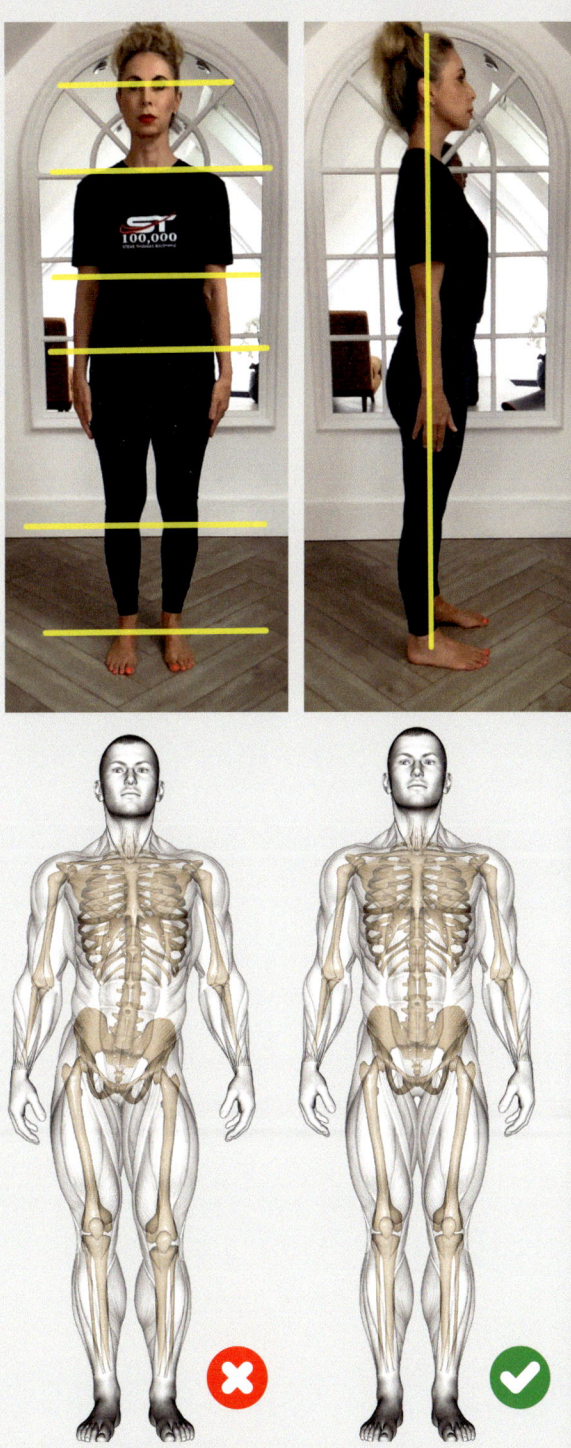

The FATHER FIGURE of FITNESS

MOVEMENT ANALYSIS

Figure 1 -
shows classic, commonplace deviations in position and movement of the feet, ankles, lower leg, knees, hips, spine and shoulders.

Figure 2 -
shows ideal skeletal alignment of the feet, ankles, lower legs, knees, hips, spine and shoulders during movement.

The consequences of Figure 2 are minimal – this is where the musculoskeletal system moves fluidly and efficiently with precision and majesty in its alignment.

The consequences of the movement patterns depicted in Figure 1 can lead to localised or isolated niggles, aches, pains and injuries or, indeed, can affect all or any combination of segments up or down throughout the body's entire kinetic chain. There are three important issues to remember here.

First, this scenario applies to the vast majority of individuals to some degree, **so it applies to you**. Second, these deviations are significant with just one stride, so jogging, running, sprinting, lifting weights, squatting, lunging – in fact any dynamic movements – exaggerate or multiply these deviations very significantly. Third, this movement pattern can result even if the initial stationary posture has good alignment – this is why x-rays and MRI scans don't always provide the required diagnosis.

Figure 1 shows clearly that when a deviated kinetic chain is set in motion it can reverberate up or down through the entire skeleton. Here we see that slight foot internal rotation (pronation) leads to internal rotation of the lower leg (tibia), which in turn leads to inward rotation of the knee (valgum), which leads to misalignment of the hips (hip drop), which leads to spinal curvature (scoliosis), which in turn leads to shoulder misalignment.

The examples shown in chapter 7 will highlight these

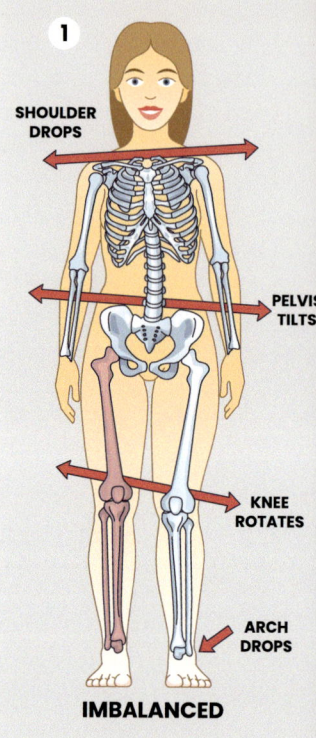

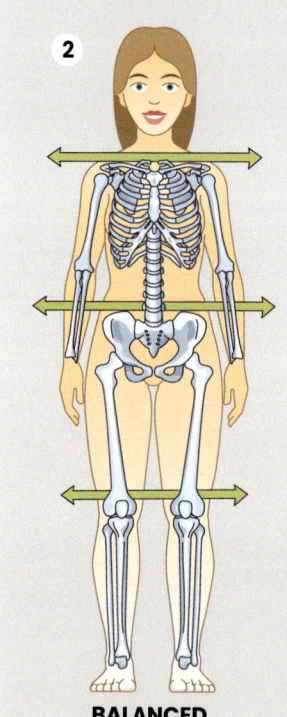

MOVEMENT ANALYSIS

issues further. Each one of these misaligned joints or segments requires significant exercise to manage or realign them. My 100,000 exercise system has all of these essential exercises built into each and every programme design.

Each joint or segment is so important that we should analyse this commonplace movement pattern in closer detail.

First, let's consider our feet and ankles. The illustration below depicts the different foot/ankle positions that the human body adopts in stance and in movement (pronation, normal/neutral, supination).

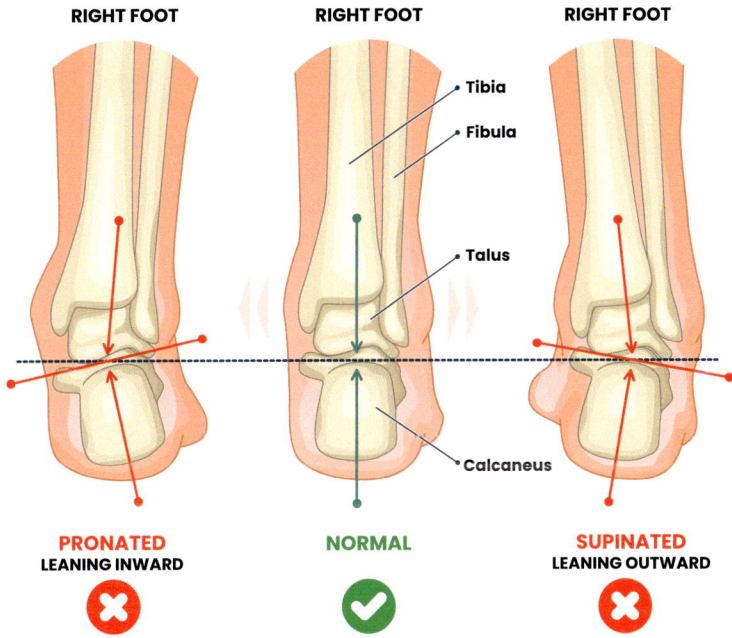

The optimal position for stance, all movement, sports and exercising is, of course, neutral. Neutral foot position and foot contact allow for smooth, balanced, fluid, efficient and controlled movement. They provide great stability and are a great starting point for the human kinetic chain.

Small deviations in pronation and/or supination can sometimes be compensated for as ground impact forces flow up through the rest of the kinetic chain. Some individuals, however, are not so fortunate. Sometimes small deviations, and certainly larger ones, put great strain on the small or delicate bones, muscles, ligaments and tendons in the feet and ankles, causing significant inflammatory pain and/or injury. Foot Levelers has said: "99 per cent of the population over-

MOVEMENT ANALYSIS

pronate to some degree". While this figure isn't universally agreed, it is quite evident that a very high percentage of individuals do over-pronate.

While over-supination is also responsible for significant musculoskeletal problems, it is not quite as prevalent as over-pronation. Indeed, my observations from many years of experience concur with a very high percentage of pronators. The effects of pronation and over-pronation are very often exacerbated by repeated movement patterns like walking, jogging, running, climbing, squatting and lunging. It is therefore a major consideration for almost every exerciser or sportsperson.

Again, slow motion video analysis is needed to observe the smallest of deviations away from neutral. If there is any small deviation(s) on either or both feet/ankles and you are experiencing **any** symptoms, then you must adhere to the foot and ankle rehabilitation exercises recommended in my 100,000 system. These exercises will address the stability, strength and balance dimensions needed to manage poor foot mechanics.

If you have significant deviation(s) on one or both feet, whether you are currently experiencing symptoms or not, I recommend a visit to a podiatrist, a specialist who specialises in foot mechanics, analysing position and movement in fine detail. If necessary, the podiatrist will manufacture orthotics: these are bespoke insoles or inlays that correct for position and function, to realign your feet and ankles.

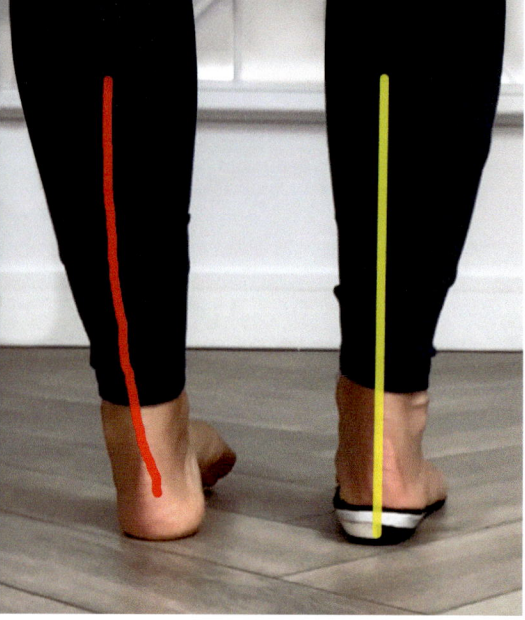

This photograph details the concept of orthotics for over-supination.

Supination as defined by orthoticsbypost.com is "commonly a result of genetics but can also be triggered or worsened by muscle imbalances in the foot, ankle and lower leg. Improper footwear, former injuries and repetitive stress lead to muscle disparity and misalignment in the body."

MOVEMENT ANALYSIS

Over-pronation frequently causes overuse-type injuries like plantar fasciitis, shin splints, bunions and spurs, which occur in repetitive movements like jogging or running. As orthoticsbypost.com also notes: "Excessive pronation, if untreated, can lead to degenerative wear and tear and chronic pain in the feet, ankles, knees, hips and spine."

The illustration here details the concept of orthotics for over-pronation.

Good alignment of feet and ankles is vitally important for human biomechanics as it affects not only the feet and ankles directly but the whole kinetic chain, rebalancing the entire musculoskeletal system. Good foot/ankle rehabilitation exercises are therefore crucial, and sometimes need to be used in conjunction with bespoke orthotics, as shown in the below photo.

The importance of 'good' or 'correct' shoes

It is imperative at this juncture to highlight the value and importance of good or correct footwear. As I have stated, orthotics or inlays are often a vital part of the realignment of an individual's feet and ankles and, hence, their entire biomechanical chain.

Logically then, good, correct stability footwear is just as important in establishing a stable base for the human body to function efficiently. All too often, 'fashion' shoes or trainers can be utterly detrimental to your mechanics. Soft, flat, fashion-led trainers are nothing short of a disaster for your feet.

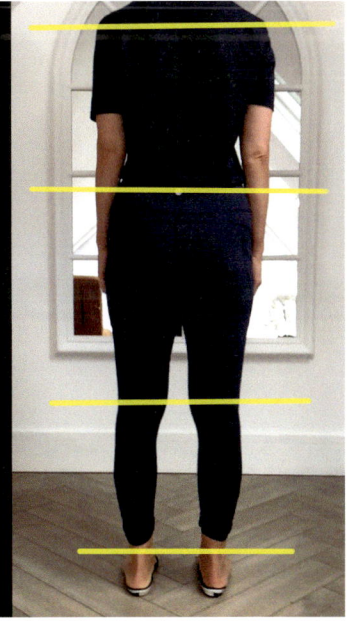

The FATHER FIGURE of FITNESS

MOVEMENT ANALYSIS

The sport shoe companies spend millions researching, designing and developing designing stability exercise and sport shoes that have great anti-pronation/anti-supination and shock-absorbency properties.

While it doesn't always follow that the most expensive shoes are the best shoes, it's important to invest in good exercise or running shoes to provide the basis for good biomechanical support. This is an issue that I see in abundance, and I encourage every one of you to understand the importance of good shoes for exercising, and indeed for general daily use. Below is an example of the importance of stability footwear.

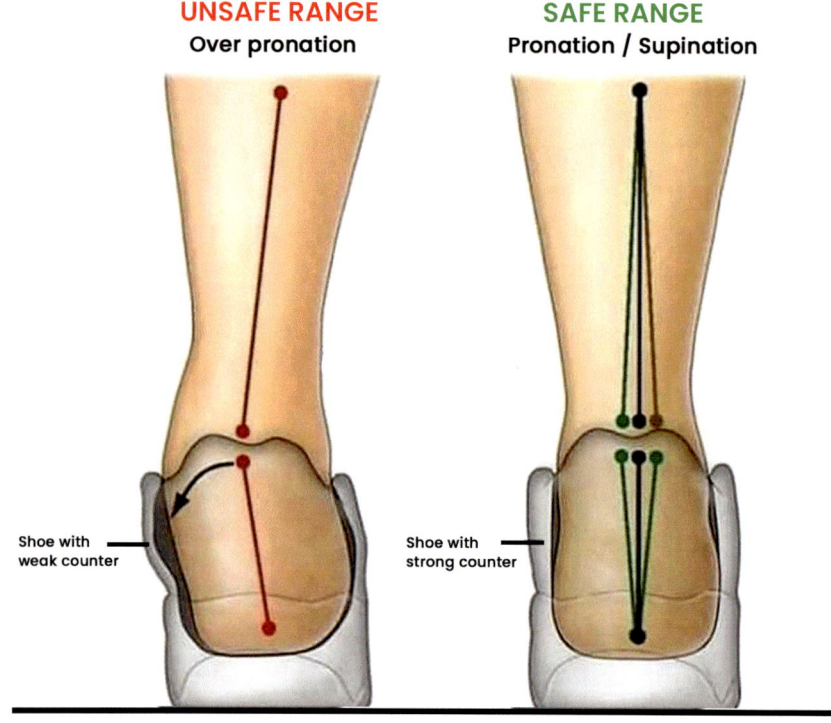

RIGHT FOOT

The next link or joint in the chain is the knee joint. Physiopedia explains: "The knee joint is one of the largest and most complex joints in the body. It is constructed by four bones and an extensive network of ligaments and muscles."

This joint has proved to be a thorn in the flesh of many regular exercisers, sportsmen

MOVEMENT ANALYSIS

and women. As a hinge joint it doesn't seem to have been very well 'designed' for many movements. The lateral movements required, and more importantly the rotational movement requirements of many activities, exercises and sports, largely explain why the incidence of knee injuries is second only to back injuries.

It is really important, both in stance and in movement (slow motion) to analyse the relationship between the hip and thigh angle and the thigh and lower leg angle.

The illustration below is a diagrammatic representation of the normal and the often-observed bow-leg and knock-knee positions.

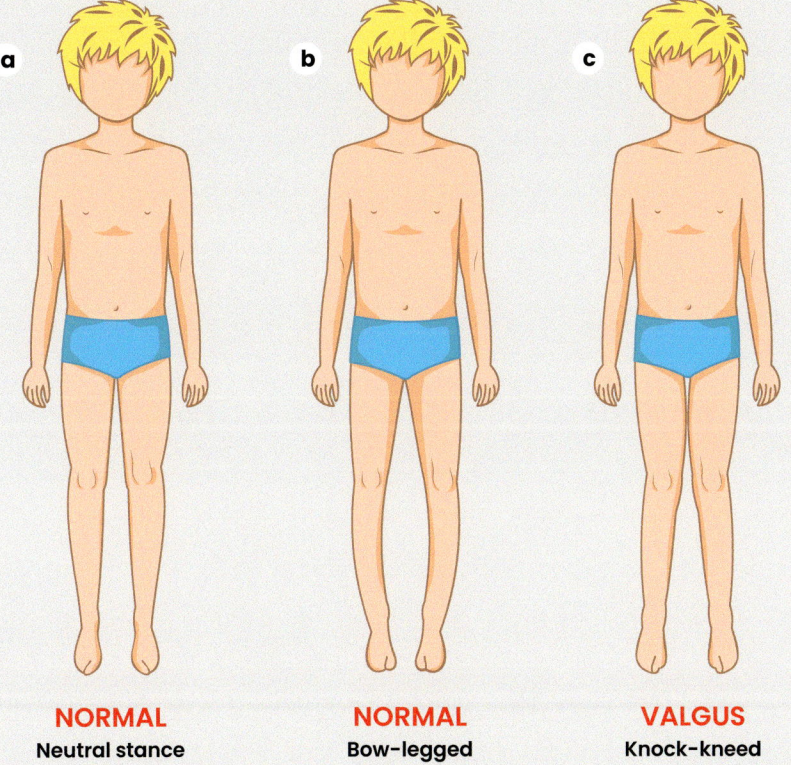

a	b	c
NORMAL	**NORMAL**	**VALGUS**
Neutral stance	Bow-legged	Knock-kneed

Position (a) above (the normal position) represents ideal leg alignment but, as I have shown and experienced many hundreds of times, this applies to a very small percentage of individuals. It's important to remember that it should not be automatically assumed that both legs function equally.

MOVEMENT ANALYSIS

In my career I have experienced all the movements patterns (a), (b) and (c) and, more importantly, varying combinations of (a), (b) and (c). This is exactly why it is so important to carry out slow-motion analysis, to see how **you** move.

My experience has shown that there simply isn't enough understanding of or respect for the knee joint, meaning there's not enough emphasis placed on it. I therefore include knee flexibility, strength, balance and stability exercises in each and every one of my 100,000 programmes.

The next joint in the human kinetic chain sequence to consider is the pelvic girdle, which itself consists of the hip joints, the sacroiliac joint and the pelvis. It's shown in the below diagram.

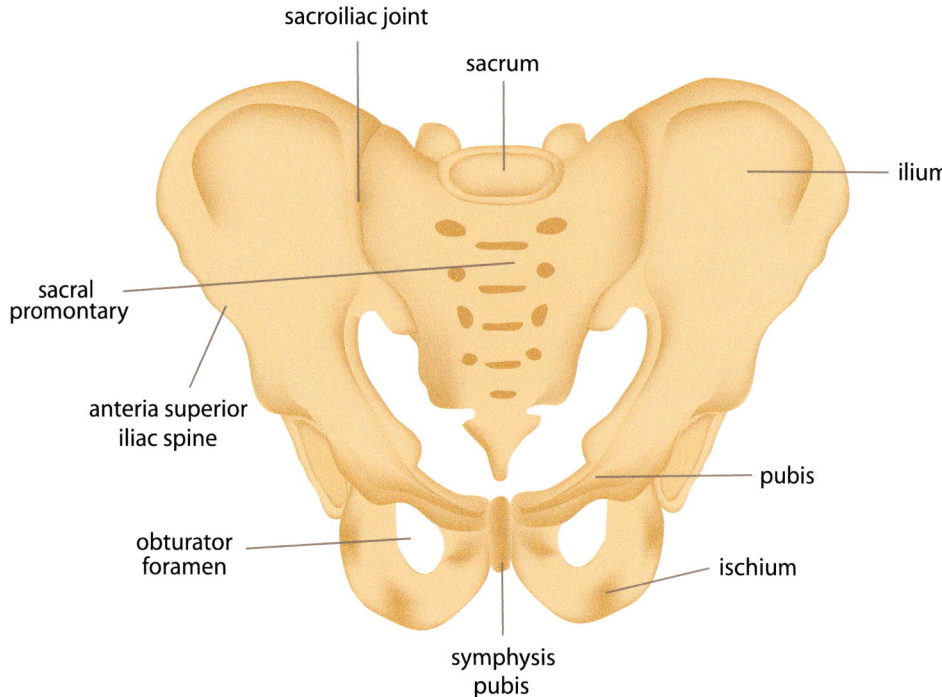

The pelvic girdle is the central 'cog' in the biomechanical chain, helping to transfer weight from the upper body and spine to the lower limbs. During gait it is also central to decreasing the forces transferred from the ground and lower extremities to the spine and upper body.

The 36 muscles of the pelvis provide stability to the joint, with a main function

MOVEMENT ANALYSIS

of *not* producing movement. Good human biomechanics is highly reliant on hip and pelvic stability and horizontal alignment. Hips and pelvic misalignment affect most individuals to some degree at some point.

The illustration below is an example of the common occurrence of hip drop (Trendelenburg gait).

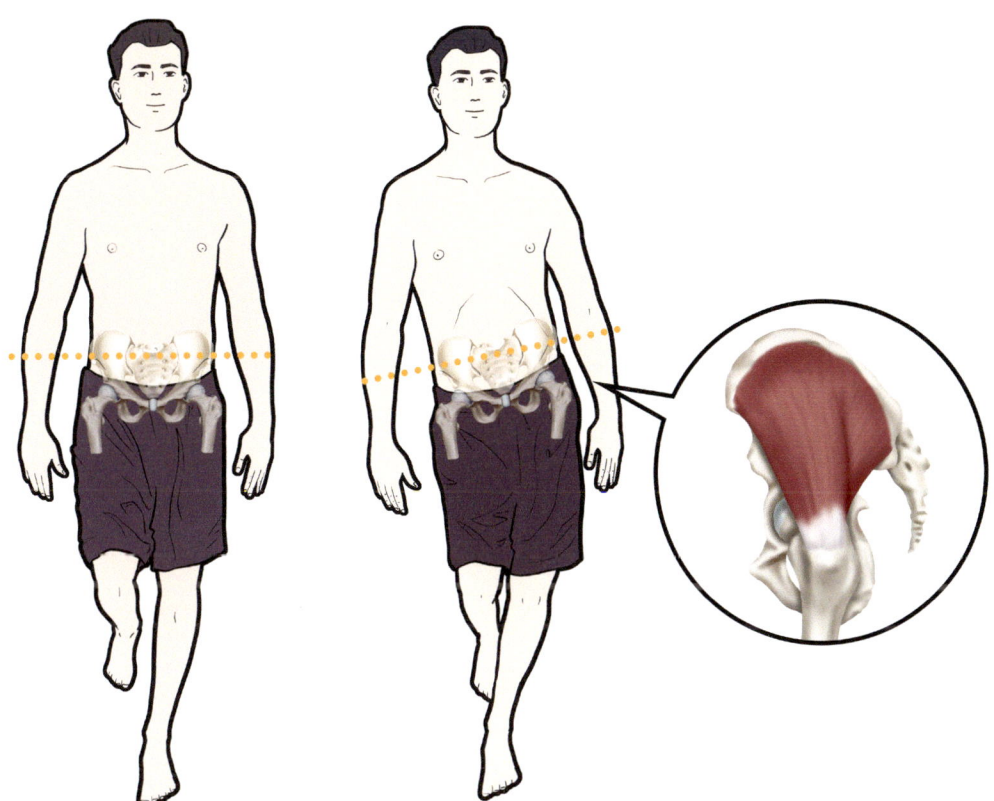

Hip drop can occur on one side or the opposite side (contralateral side), or it can be bilateral (both sides). The gluteus medius muscle is essential to the movement and mechanics of the hips and pelvis, and this is why I have flooded my 100,000 system with the best gluteal muscle exercises.

Again, slow-motion analysis is essential to study hip and pelvis angles during gait. In addition, it's imperative to analyse your slow-motion footage from a side view. The photograph below shows the various pelvic tilted positions that are also frequently observed.

MOVEMENT ANALYSIS

Is your pelvic tilt causing your back pain?

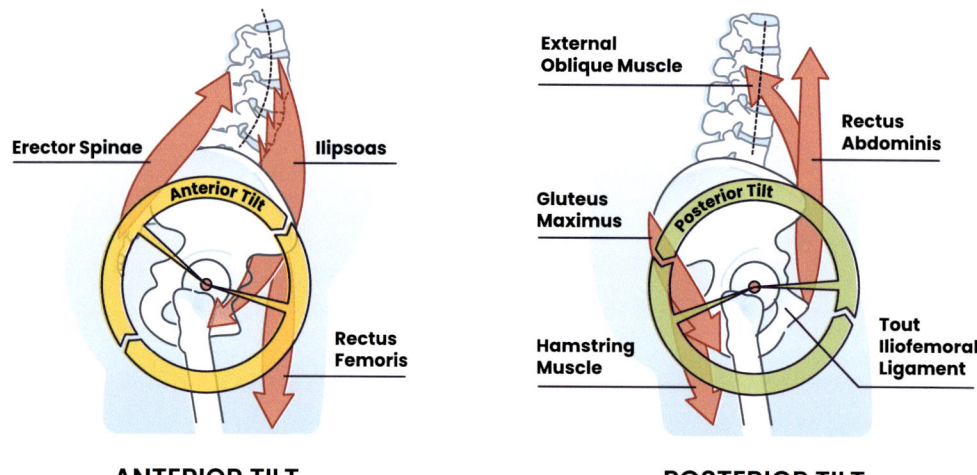

ANTERIOR TILT **POSTERIOR TILT**

Both anterior and posterior tilted positions of the pelvis during stance and movement can have very significant consequences on the musculoskeletal system. Similarly, the sacroiliac joint (SI joint) is vital in human biomechanics.

Are you, like millions of others, suffering from nagging lower back pain? Could the problem be your SI joint? The SI joint lies between the iliac bone and the sacrum, as depicted below.

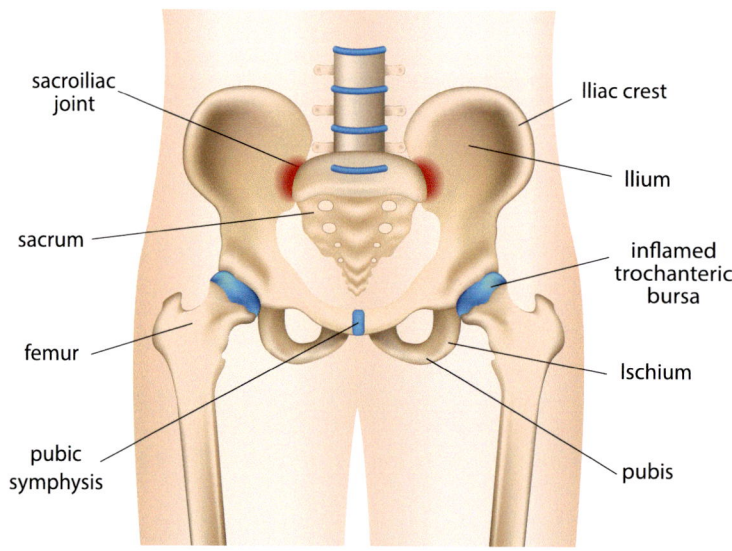

MOVEMENT ANALYSIS

Individuals with altered gait patterns, spinal curvatures and/or leg length discrepancies often experience SI joint pain, which can also result from continuous repetitive movements like squats and lunges and activities such as running, jumping and many team and individual sports. This can cause a build-up of trauma-related injuries over time.

My experience has shown me the high prevalence of SI joint pain, and I have therefore 'prescribed' high-grade stability exercises for this joint, which are vital if you are to attain and maintain fluidity of hip and pelvic function.

It is important to mention here the iliotibial (IT) band, depicted below. This is a thick band of fascia (connective tissue) that originates at the pelvis and runs down the lateral or outside of the thigh and crosses the knee joint. Inflammation of this fascia is a common issue for many runners, athletes and exercisers.

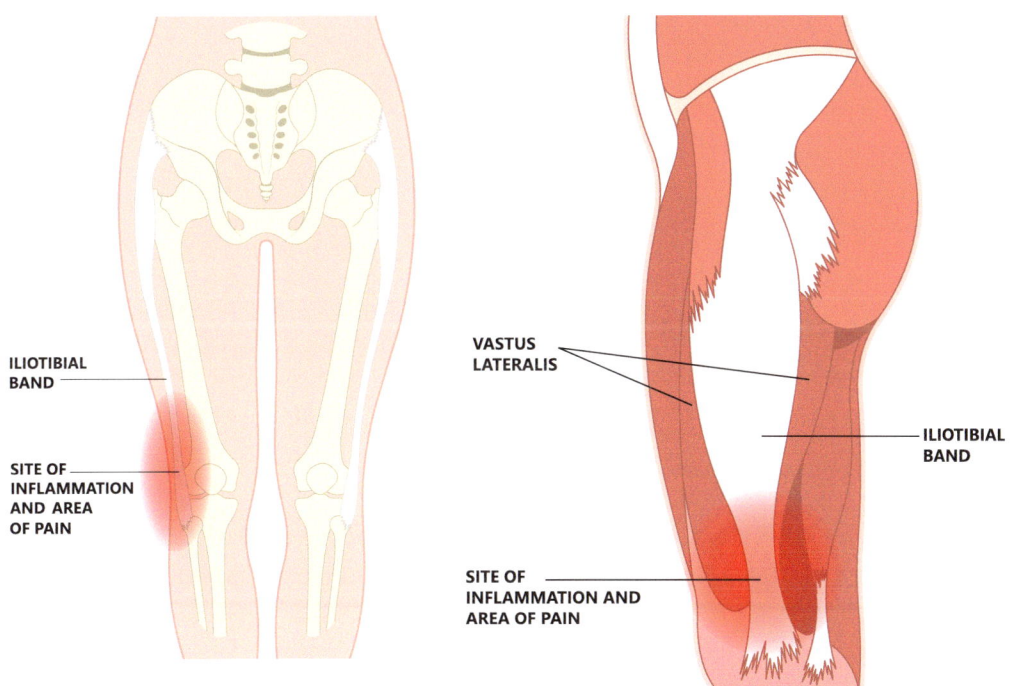

The IT band is vital for knee position and stability, and it plays a major role in many exercises, activities and sports. Iliotibial band syndrome is very common and, while it isn't diagnosed directly from slow-motion movement analysis, it is very much linked with and symptomatic of foot over-pronation and one, or both, knees collapsing inwards.

MOVEMENT ANALYSIS

Many teachers, coaches and personal trainers are now aware of the importance of the iliotibial band, but the practice of trying to release it is being carried out completely incorrectly. My 100,000 exercise programmes address this issue in every routine.

The next segment in the human kinetic chain, so crucial to the overall functioning of the human body, is the spine. I have already stated that the spinal structure and system of bones, muscles and joints is impressive, adaptable, majestic and multifunctional, and at its best it can be flexible and fluid.

Because of its complexity, however, it is also a major breeding ground for biomechanical compensations and hence problems that lead to aches, pains, injuries, surgeries and suffering. In short, THE WORLD IS FULL OF BACK PAIN.

Analysis of your slow-motion video footage needs to be well considered, careful, precise and take account of the front, side and rear views. The below illustration shows the various curvatures of which you need to be aware.

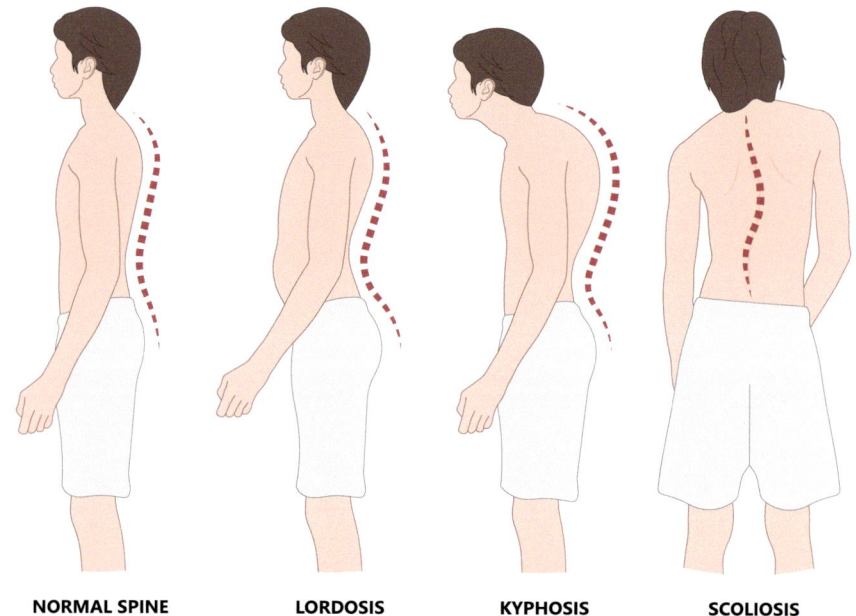

NORMAL SPINE   **LORDOSIS**   **KYPHOSIS**   **SCOLIOSIS**

The above spinal curvatures are clear and pronounced and exist even in the most athletic of individuals, but during **your** analysis of your spine you must look out for **any** deviations, however small they appear. Even minor deviations can lead, directly and/or indirectly, to major compensations and consequences.

MOVEMENT ANALYSIS

For your spine to continue to function organically and naturally, it requires many exercise components. First, it requires multifunctional flexibility and strength – this consists of a well-balanced combination of:

- Static stretching exercises.
- Dynamic stretching exercises.
- Spinal mobility exercises.
- Postural exercises.
- Abdominal/core strengthening exercises.
- Upper, middle and lower back muscle-strengthening exercises.
- Good head and neck positions and exercises.

Second, it requires foundational flexibility and strength from the hips, pelvis and gluteal musculature. This consists of a well-balanced combination of:

- Hip/pelvic mobility exercises.
- Hip/pelvic strength exercises.
- Hip/pelvic stability exercises.
- Balance/proprioception exercises.
- Gluteal strengthening exercises.

While lower and general back pain have been the bane of so many individuals' lives for many decades, a new pandemic is brewing at an alarming rate. The modern world is changing our postural habits and we are blissfully unaware. These new habits are creeping up on us and we are potentially heading for significant problems.

The below depicts the 'modern-day' phenomenon of 'tech neck'.

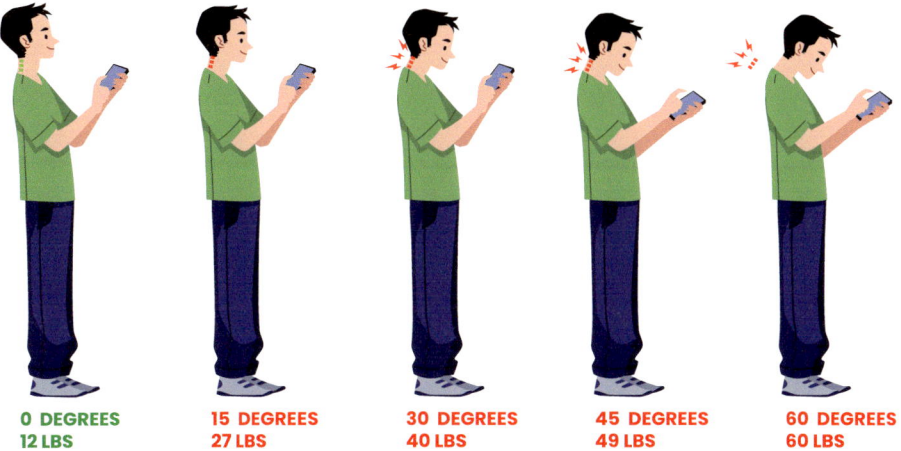

MOVEMENT ANALYSIS

Our modern-day reliance on technology and our use of computers, tablets and mobile phones is encouraging spinal and postural adaptations that will eventuate into a skeletal pandemic if they are left untreated. As the previous illustration shows, the increased weight and forces from even slight forward head position will produce significant load-bearing consequences and issues for the upper (thoracic) spine.

These consequences are being stored up and must be addressed now, or these loads will damage the spine and cause ongoing issues down through the middle back and into the lower spine – or, indeed, the entire human kinetic chain.

A multifaceted approach is therefore needed for spinal health and fitness. Follow my comprehensive 100,000 system and you will flood your spine with 'nutrient'-dense exercises – you will feed it, you will respect it and you will look after it. More importantly, it will look after you.

Even before the modern phenomenon of 'tech neck', the upper spine, neck and shoulders were the forgotten segments in exercise regimes. Routines rich in exercises for the head and neck position and posture and exercises for upper spine (thoracic) mobility and for shoulder joint and shoulder girdle position, posture and impingement syndrome have been non-existent. Bad postural habits, technology, incorrect pillows and mattresses, psychological stress, heavy weightlifting, incorrect exercise selection, poor exercise technique and bad trends in exercise have all had major consequences for the upper spine, neck and shoulders.

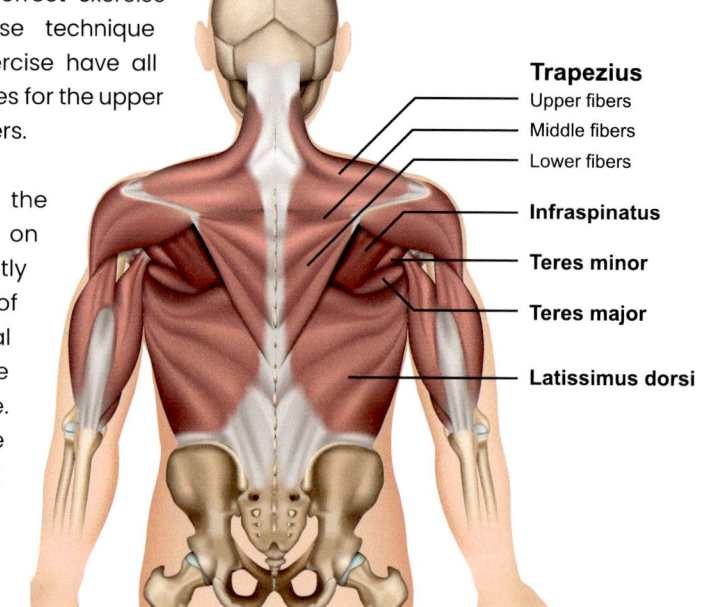

This explains why the shoulder joint is third on the list of most frequently operated on areas of the musculoskeletal system, behind the knee joint and the back/spine. The illustration here shows the complex array of muscles in the upper back, neck and shoulders.

MOVEMENT ANALYSIS

The anatomy of the upper spine, neck and shoulders shows a very complex network of bones, joints, muscles, tendon, ligaments and nerves that must all function with intricate precision of movements, coordination and timing to prevent problematic compensations. The shoulder joint alone has multiple overlapping muscles and tissue, all functioning in a very small space and hence with very little room for manoeuvre. Shoulder impingement syndrome, frozen shoulder, neck tightness and upper spine postural problems are all too common.

There are many popular regular exercises that **you** simply should **not** perform, and many others that you **must** start to practise immediately. These exercises are fully explained in Chapter 8, Development of my 100,000 system.

Upper spine, head, neck and shoulders require precise and special attention with a well-balanced, well-executed combination of postural, joint mobility, flexibility and muscular strengthening exercises, especially for the rotator cuff musculature (supraspinatus, infraspinatus, subscapularis and teres major), which my exercise system will deliver.

In summary, the fundamental missing link in the world of health, fitness and personal exercise is:

HUMAN BIOMECHANICS and HUMAN MOVEMENT.

Whatever your age, height, weight, experience, fitness or performance level, and whatever your goals or objectives are, understanding **your** posture, how **you** stand and how **you** walk and move is vitally important in establishing what exercise **you** should do. So my **Golden Rule Number Four** – taking video footage and analysing **your** gait – is vital.

The following examples show clearly why an understanding of biomechanics, posture and movement is so important for each and every one of us. They will allow you to visualise and understand how and why I have developed these methods, and why I use them with my personal clients. They are genuine examples of clients, individuals who, without slow-motion analysis and a full understanding of their movement patterns, would have ended up following completely wrong exercise routines.

Follow my methods and you can learn why my 100,000 system will allow you to progress faster than ever, bullet-proofing your musculoskeletal system and exercising with much greater efficiency. It really is the FUTURE OF EXERCISE.

MOVEMENT ANALYSIS

Example 1

The photo is of a young woman in her normal 'stationary' stance position. **What do you see?**

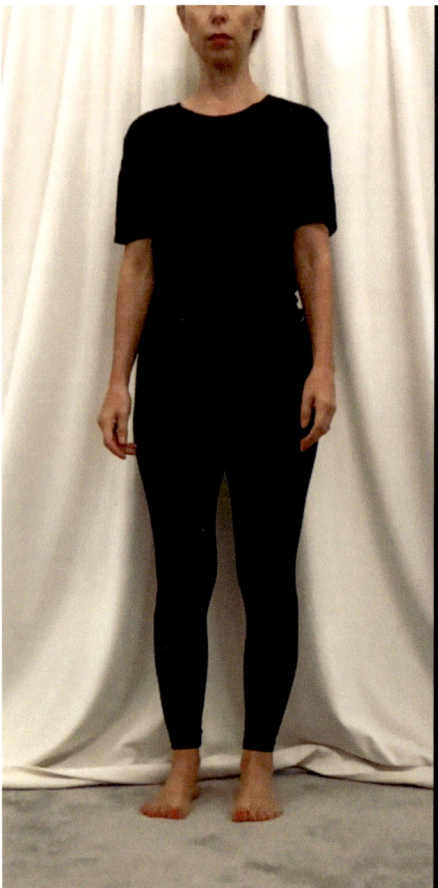

Visual analysis reveals a young, fit, slim, lean, healthy, well-proportioned, athletic individual with good posture. Add to this her physical details:

– Height – 5ft 5in
– Weight – 8.5 stone
– Clothes – size 8 (UK)
– Non-smoker
– Non-drinker
– Low resting heart rate
– Low/average blood pressure
– Low cholesterol
– Very healthy diet
– Medical history completely clear
– Very low body fat percentage

Add to this her weekly exercise routine:

– 20 to 40 minutes running four to six days a week
– 40-minute gym sessions four to five days a week

I'm sure you would conclude, as would most coaches, teachers, doctors and personal trainers, that this individual is visually, nutritionally and medically in great shape, very fit, strong and in great health.

By all current medical and health and fitness professionals' standards, this individual would be given the green light, encouraged to participate in almost **any** exercise routines or regimes she liked. Surely she could benefit from high-intensity or low-intensity training, dynamic training, static training, fast movements, slow

MOVEMENT ANALYSIS

movements, compound movements, isolation movements – in fact, any training regimes or routines that have ever been developed. But is this the case?

The above information is of course, very important, but THIS IS NOT WHAT I SEE.

My sport science background, knowledge and experience tell me that the above information, despite being important, is simply not enough. This is where the whole exercising world is getting things wrong.

Designing a traditional exercise routine for this individual would almost certainly lead to disaster.

1. Walking, jogging, running – **completely wrong**.
2. Lunging (stationary or walking) – **completely wrong**.
3. Deep squatting – **completely wrong**.
4. Sprinting – **completely wrong**.
5. Press-ups – **completely wrong**.
6. Pull-ups – **completely wrong**.
7. Full sit-ups – **completely wrong**.
8. Plank – **completely wrong**.
9. High intensity training – **completely wrong**.
10. Heavy weight training – **completely wrong**.
11. Many yoga positions – **completely wrong**.
12. Rowing machines – **completely wrong.**
13. Stepper machines – **completely wrong.**
14. Side bends – **completely wrong.**
15. Boxing – **completely wrong.**
16. Most dynamic sports – **completely wrong.**

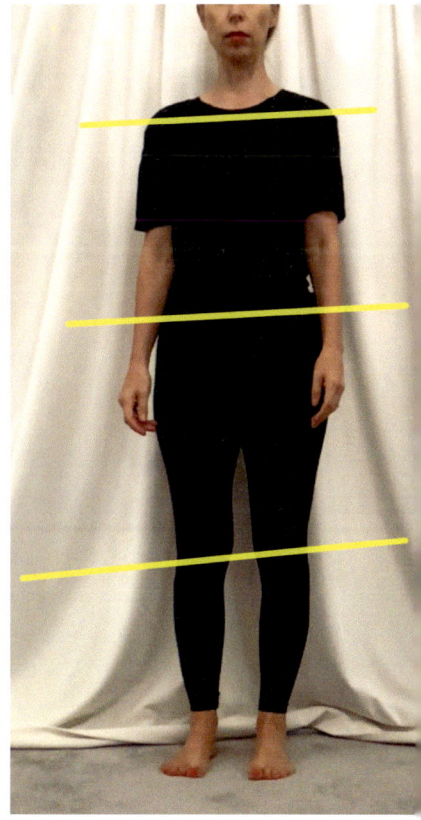

Even though this list isn't exhaustive, you must be wondering why I wouldn't prescribe what are regarded as normal, basic, even 'staple' exercises for this fit and healthy individual. Let me explain.

THIS IS WHAT I SEE (photo right):

- Shoulder misalignment
- Hip/pelvic misalignment
- Knee joint misalignment

Even though this individual is completely stationary,

MOVEMENT ANALYSIS

these misalignment issues are red flags, and I am already suspicious that there may exist significant musculoskeletal compensations. Further exploration is needed. This is where slow-motion movement analysis is crucial.

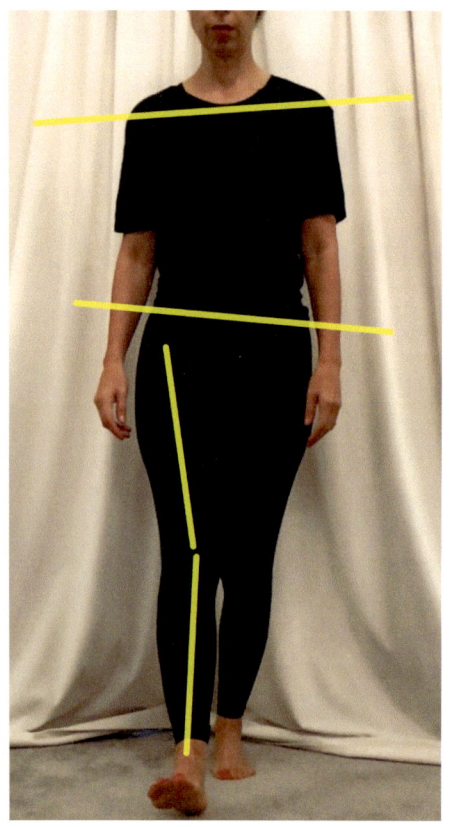

Even during the first stride of my slow-motion movement analysis (front view), my suspicions are confirmed. As the right foot (heel) contacts the ground we see an all-too-familiar musculoskeletal pattern of movement. The right foot 'rolls' inward (over-pronation); this forces the lower leg to rotate internally (internal rotation); this in turn causes knee valgum (knock knees); this leads to the wrong angle (collapsing inwards) of the thigh bone (femur).

This part of the full chain of movement alone can put tremendous extra strain on the foot, ankle, knee and hip/pelvis.

The photo (left) also clearly shows that as the right leg extends (straightens), taking the individual's body weight, the opposite (left) hip falls away, clearly showing that the hips and pelvis are not horizontal. To ensure that the eyes stay horizontal, and the whole body does not collapse to the left, the right shoulder drops further than in a stationary stance position, to counterbalance the bodyweight. Again, here the shoulders are not horizontal.

It is clear to see that the resulting angles of both the hips/pelvis and the shoulders can only produce one consequence for the spine (back): it puts it in a completely incorrect and unstable position. The spine can only relax and function smoothly and correctly when it has a horizontal, stable platform to sit on, below and level/in horizontal alignment with the shoulders, above.

The example shows the **opposite** of good, correct, ideal spinal position. The predicted consequence of these movement patterns is **compensation** – and

MOVEMENT ANALYSIS

please remember that this is the consequence of just one stride. This individual's musculoskeletal system is overworking and being overloaded at each and every stride, trying to compensate at each and every link in the movement chain, to try to maintain the upright, correct, vertical postural alignment that the skeleton craves in order to continue to work and function fluently, efficiently and majestically.

Slow-motion movement analysis from the rear view (Photo below) only serves to confirm these findings – the pattern of movement is repetitive with each and every stride.

This rear view again shows poor, inefficient biomechanics (body movements):

– **Inefficient foot position**
– **Inefficient lower leg position**
– **Inefficient knee position**
– **Inefficient hip/pelvis position**

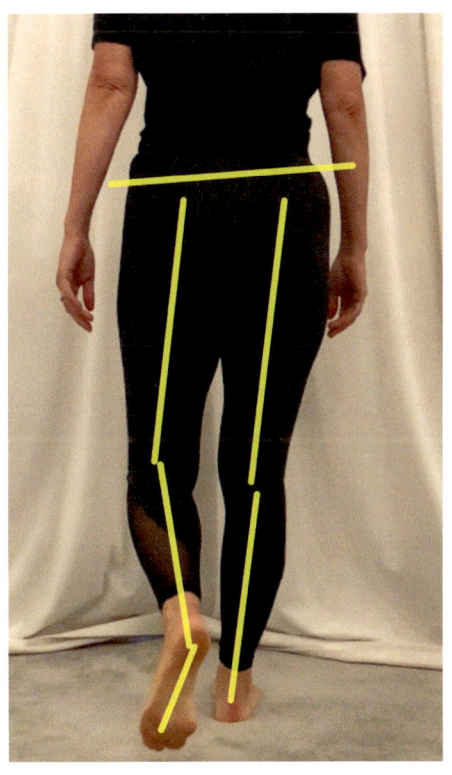

Without the ideal, correct postural alignment, and hence fluid movement, the body will begin to tighten and tighten and tighten, until niggles, aches and pains begin to appear.

Without the correct intervention with bespoke exercise prescription to bulletproof these musculoskeletal inefficiencies, this individual may be heading for a lifetime of frustration, pain and injury. Her current exercising routine may be making her worse and not better. This is a situation that, as I have explained, is all too commonplace in a world where the exercising culture is booming.

Further investigation for this individual revealed a 6mm structural leg length discrepancy, and equally importantly, a ten-year history of constant frustration, pain and injury, exactly as predicted.

Even though she is fit and healthy visually, nutritionally and medically, biomechanics analysis has been the missing link. Without this, this individual

MOVEMENT ANALYSIS

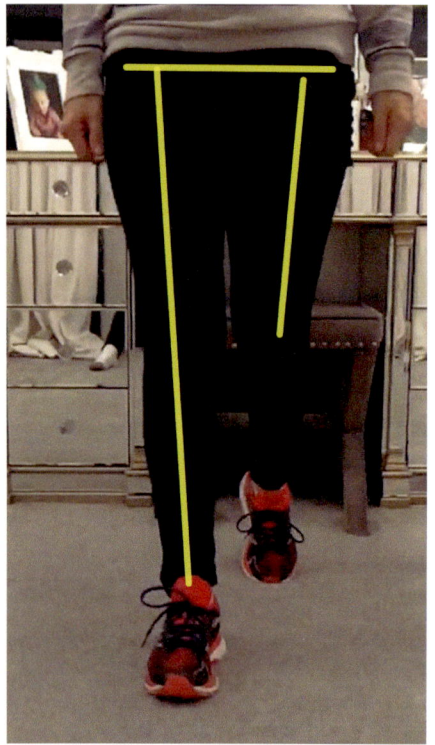

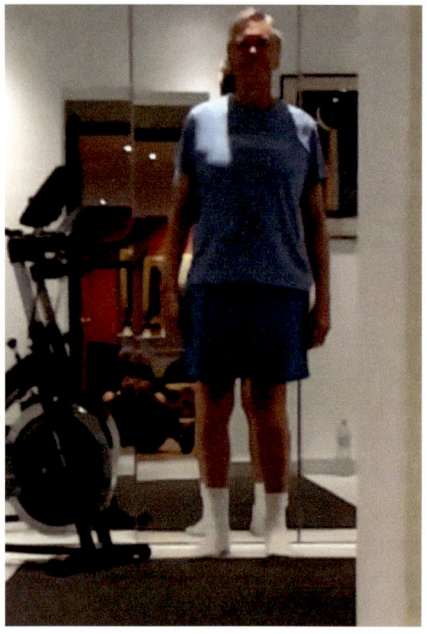

has suffered hip, pelvis and lower back pain, upper back pain, neck pain and headaches, sciatic and other nerve pain, early-onset scoliosis and sacroiliac joint pain for over ten years. Despite many x-rays and MRI scans, and an enormous amount of treatment, her discomfort and pain continued.

I prescribed my 100,000 exercise system for her, along with a visit to leading UK podiatrist Trevor Prior, who designed bespoke orthotics, insoles and inlays, to promote foot position and correct for her 6mm leg length issue.

I was confident that we eventually had this individual working on the correct exercise routines to address these issues, but it still required a lot of time, work and effort. I can report that she is back running four to six sessions a week, is significantly structurally fitter and stronger and, more importantly, **completely pain-free**. The photo (above left) clearly shows the significant improvement in her biomechanics. The leg alignment is perfect, as is the hip/pelvic alignment.

Let's take a look at another example.

This is my great friend and client Charles Delevingne (photo left), father of Chloe, Poppy and Cara. He is tall (6ft 3in) with a strong, athletic physique, and plays golf and tennis and shoots. The photograph left shows a front view of Charles in his normal stationary stance.

What do you see?

MOVEMENT ANALYSIS

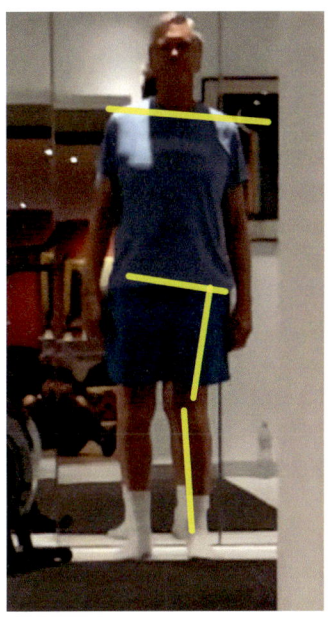

At first glance one would be forgiven for not seeing anything out of the ordinary. However, this is **what I see**:

Look at both the shoulder and hip/pelvis alignment, and indeed the stationary leg positions. Even during these stationary standing positions, the whole body appears to be collapsing away on the left side. These issues again are red flags, showing complete lop-sidedness of the entire musculoskeletal system. Even prior to movement analysis I have a strong inclination that there exist significant knee, hip, pelvis, spine, neck and/or shoulder issues.

The photographs below show Charles' movement mechanics.

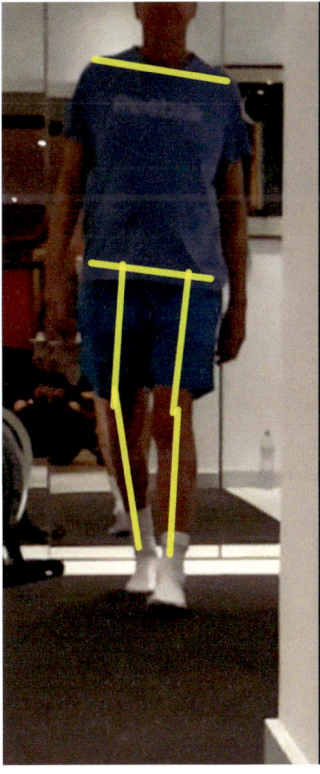

As I suspected, during right foot floor contact, the whole of Charles's body collapses away on his left side, with the misalignment of the shoulders and hips being even more pronounced than in the stationary position. The photograph right (rear view) also reveals that Charles's right hip falls away (hip drop) as his left foot contacts the ground.

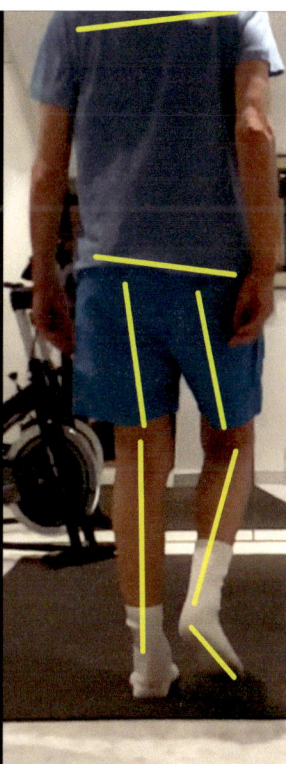

MOVEMENT ANALYSIS

Further investigation uncovered a small but significant (4mm) leg length discrepancy, poor foot mechanics and, more importantly, a long history of knee, hip, pelvis, lower back, middle back, upper back, neck and shoulder tightness and significant pain. X-rays also revealed very significant spinal curvature (scoliosis). Shooting, playing tennis and golf with these musculoskeletal inefficiencies would eventually lead to disaster.

Prescribing traditional exercise routines would be **completely wrong**; traditional gym exercises would be **completely wrong**; high-intensity training, dynamic movement exercises and various sports would be **completely wrong**.

Just attempting to get fitter and stronger in the traditional exercising manner simply won't work. This again is why so many exercisers are getting worse and not better. The wrong exercise prescription here would again exacerbate these areas of tightness, the niggles, aches and pains – in essence we would continue on a fast track to pain, injury and potential surgery.

What Charles needs is full biomechanical support, bespoke exercise prescription that is packed with foot, ankle, knee, hip, pelvis, spine, neck and shoulder stability exercises, spinal mobility exercises, nerve stretches, static and dynamic stretching, postural realignment exercises and orthotics for correction of foot mechanics.

As his personal trainer, I have prescribed my 100,000 exercise system and we are working to change, rectify and stabilise all of these issues. Our goal, of course, is to be completely pain-free, stabilise and bulletproof the entire body and become fitter, stronger, and healthier.

I can report that he is responding remarkably quickly, and we are well on our way to achieving our goals. I may even one day let him beat me on the tennis court (only joking). The correct exercise prescription will realign, re-educate, almost restructure the musculoskeletal system, regaining the stability, fluidity, flexibility and mobility that every one of us needs to flourish, progress and reach our goals.

There is no denying that achieving full body realignment takes time, hard work, patience and dedication, but the results can be spectacular.

I have chosen these two examples as they both show an almost entire body (kinetic) chain reaction – from foot contact right through the whole body to the head, neck and shoulders – and they are both quite pronounced. For educational

MOVEMENT ANALYSIS

purposes, they are perfect examples of what we need to be aware of, and how essential it is for each and every one of us to analyse our own movement patterns. After all, this is what makes you, you, and it is what **must** underpin all of your exercise choices.

It's important to state that I've not had to look far and wide for these examples; they're not unique – they are in fact, all too commonplace. I have literally thousands of examples. Many individuals just have isolated issues at one point or another in the full kinetic chain; more importantly, they may only be seemingly insignificant misalignments, but even very small misalignments *must* be addressed, as they will almost certainly develop into greater issues.

Remember, without slow-motion (biomechanical) analysis it is almost impossible to see these misalignment patterns. It's **imperative** that we all analyse our movements in slow motion.

This is exactly why slow-motion analysis is one of my **golden rules**, and why my 100,000 system, consisting of all the various components needed to address these multi-segmental issues, has been developed.

We have established that efficient human musculoskeletal movement patterns can be majestic in its capabilities, but we have also established that it is nothing short of miraculous to have or achieve this. This dictates that every one of us has a biomechanical pattern that needs close inspection and close attention.

In short, every one of us needs bespoke, varied and detailed exercise routines to address the flexibility, fluidity, stability, balance and strength of each of the body's segments – feet, ankles, knees, hips, pelvis, spine, head, neck and shoulders – in isolation and the flexibility, fluidity, stability, balance and strength of the human kinetic chain as a whole.

This concludes that **you** have musculoskeletal issues that are holding you back – issues that you must understand, respect and deal with. It's so important to understand and realise the enormous influence – the power, almost – that correct, varied, balanced and well-executed exercises can have on the human body.

The body is quite remarkable at ironing problems out and rectifying a multitude of issues when it is given the correct variety and balance of exercises. But we must encourage it, nurse it and smother it in beautifully well-crafted, well-oiled, varied and fluid exercises and movements. When we do this, it will respond as

MOVEMENT ANALYSIS

it never has before, banishing your niggles, aches and pains, increasing your stability, recovering from your injuries and bullet-proofing your musculoskeletal system, allowing it to perform, flourish and produce unbelievable results.

This has been my lifelong work: making **your** exercise about **you** – efficient, effective and productive.

Development of my 100,000 system

Throughout my career I have had the great privilege of working closely with some of the world's biggest stars and many individuals from all over the world who have had wide experience of different exercise philosophies and worked with many coaches, teachers and personal trainers.

My philosophy, motivation and driving force has always been focused on bringing science into exercise and making it personal and bespoke, designed for every individual. My methods have always started with the individual client and his or her body, his or her skeleton – analysing their stance, their gait and their movement and building their personal exercise programmes based on this analysis.

As time went on I started to receive wonderful feedback from clients, often being called "the best personal trainer in the UK", even "the best personal trainer in the world". This feedback was very flattering, but it only served to highlight that I was doing things differently and that good scientific, bespoke exercise advice was simply not getting through to the population at large.

I was realising that most people were still following out-of-date ideas and principles, even though our scientific knowledge and understanding of the human body, its biomechanics and its compensatory patterns had advanced immeasurably. I was seeing so much that was wrong, so much that needed to change, and I knew that I had the answers.

So I have felt an enormous weight of responsibility, a sense of duty, to pass on my knowledge and experience, so that **you** can change **your** approach, **your** attitude and **your** perspective on how **you** should exercise.

My challenge, therefore, has been to overcome the multitude of issues, problems and mistakes that everyone makes, and incorporate the multitude of missing components necessary into developing a comprehensive, detailed, varied, universal system from which **everyone** can learn and progress.

DEVELOPMENT OF MY 100,000 SYSTEM

I needed to develop a regime loaded with my **top tips** and the secrets that I have developed and utilised, tried and tested thousands of times, so that you can exercise better and smarter, with full consideration of your biomechanics, attaining and retaining your majestic, fluid, flexible, strong and robust musculoskeletal system and ensuring fast and efficient results.

The exercise/fitness world has become a magnet for fashionable exercises, positions and movements, and therefore, as my first port of call, I needed to address some of the most common *mistakes* – the things that **everyone** is getting wrong. Are **you** one of the millions of people who do any or all of the following?

1. The plank

Let's start with the exercise that most epitomises my challenge – the modern-day phenomenon that is the plank.

This exercise has somehow swept through the fitness world as if it were the holy grail of all exercises. If we simply continue to follow all the exercise trends as we have for over 37 years, we should all bow down to this miraculous masterpiece of an exercise.

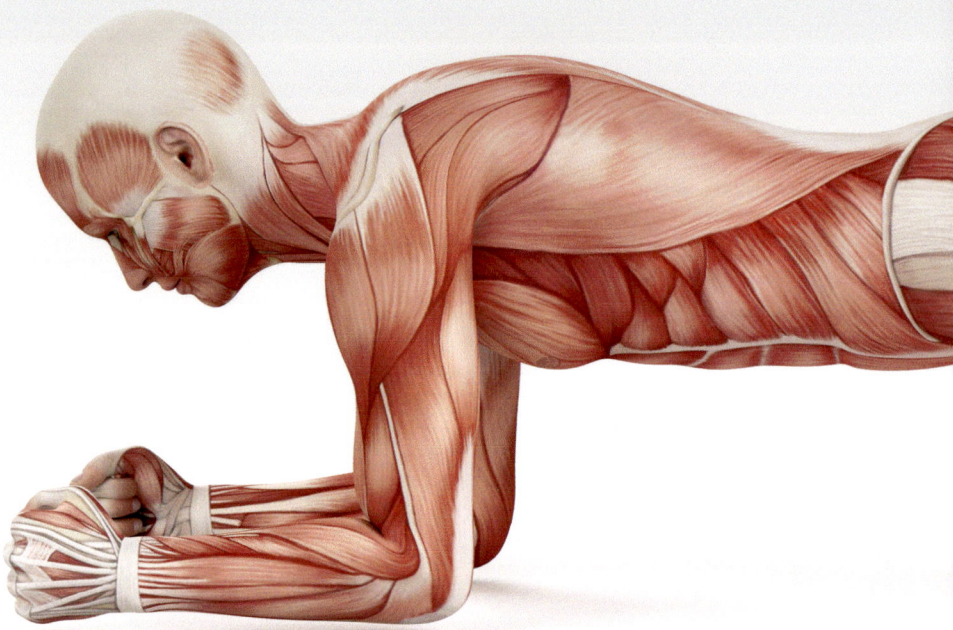

DEVELOPMENT OF MY 100,000 SYSTEM

The exact origins of the plank are not known; however, Joseph Pilates invented and used a plankesque movement in the 1920s. Royal H Burpee, who introduced burpees in the 1930s/1940s incorporated a plank element into the exercise. Irrespective of its origin, the plank has become a status symbol for anyone who can hold the position for more than five minutes. There are regular plank-offs and even a world record that currently stands at 9 hours 38 minutes and 47 seconds.

As a sport scientist, however, I see it differently. Let's look at the scientific detail of this exercise a bit more closely.

The image below represents the plank.

This static/isometric exercise is very much in vogue, being a 'must do' in all modern exercise routines. I would go as far as to say that the whole exercise world seems to have become obsessed with the plank, believing that it is simply the best position or exercise that we should all do. Is it really the amazing must-do exercise that we've been brainwashed to believe in?

As a sport scientist, my simple answer is **no**. It is probably the most over-performed and under– delivering exercise of all. Is it even doing what we believe it's doing? **No**.

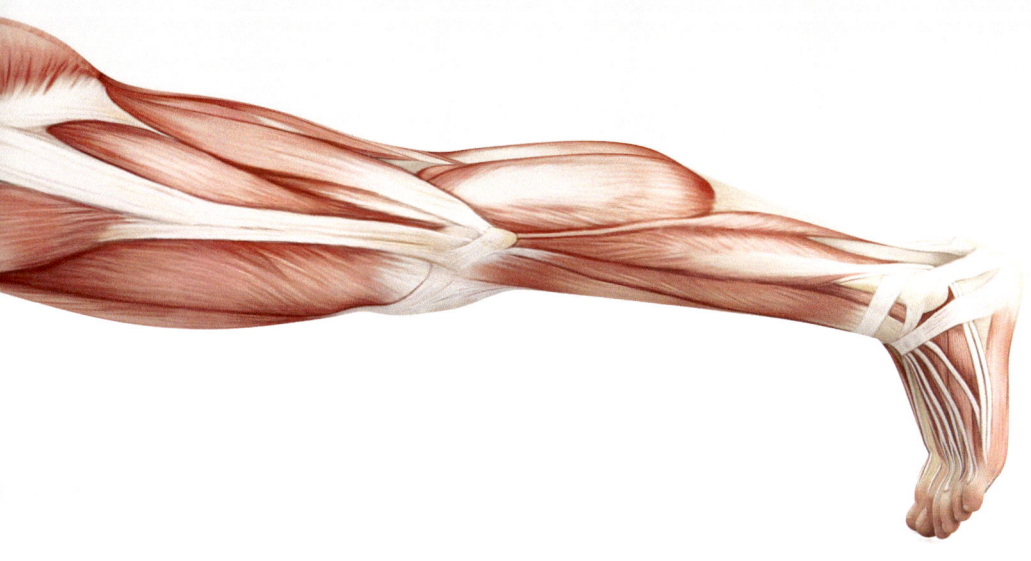

DEVELOPMENT OF MY 100,000 SYSTEM

You have probably heard or been taught that the traditional plank is the best exercise for:

1. Your core. *This simply isn't true.*

Do we fully understand what core stability really means? No: your body's core is not just your abdominal area, technically it is your lumbar, pelvic and hip region. This is collectively known as the lumbopelvic hip complex (LPHC). Optimal core training also needs to involve rotational trunk mobility and stability exercises, and this traditional position just does not deliver this.

2. Your posture. *This is also simply not true – in fact, the opposite may apply.*

This position relies on isometric shoulder protraction (pulling the shoulders forward) and not shoulder retraction (pulling the shoulders backwards), which would be necessary for better posture.

3. Your lower back. *This is incorrect.*

The traditional plank relies heavily on isometric hip flexor (upper thigh) activity. Too much hip flexor contraction can pull the pelvis forward into an anterior tilted position, encouraging a curved, concave lower spine position – a counterproductive position for correct spinal posture.

4. Your glutes. *Even if you actively 'squeeze' your glutes, they are not contracting against any load, therefore not producing any significant benefit.*

So spending minutes, even hours, in this simple, one-dimensional, isometric suspended position simply does not do it – it is seriously **over-rated**.

It is important to understand that every time you do a plank you are tensing the intercostal muscles between the ribs and the pectoral (chest) muscles. This puts pressure on the costochondral joint – the area of cartilage joining the ribs to the breastbone. This can sometimes cause inflammation (costochondritis; see diagram opposite), which is very painful and not as uncommon as you may think.

If this is you, STOP DOING IT– STOP WASTING YOUR TIME.

It's imperative to note that if you have joint instability or loose ligaments (hypermobility), I would recommend that you never do the plank.

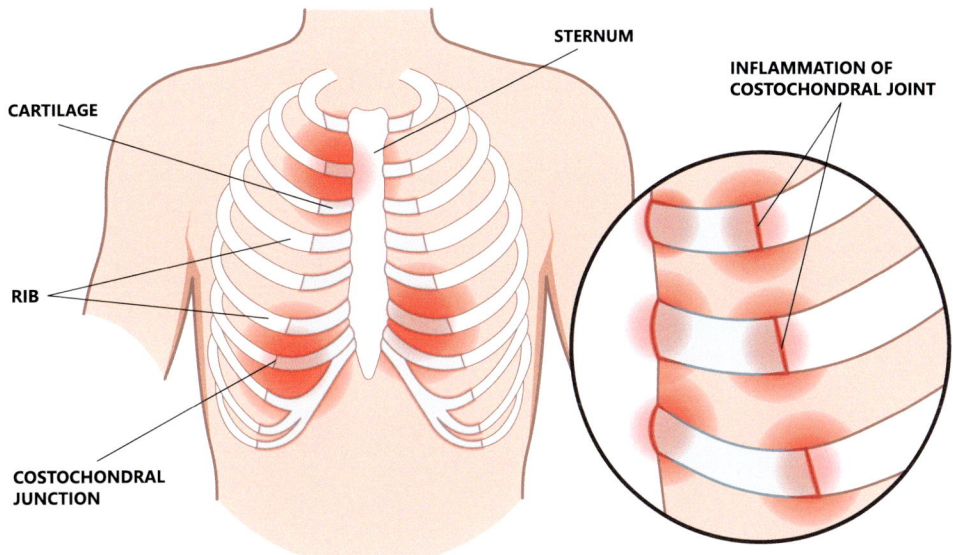

In summary, whilst there are no 'bad' exercises, and the eminent back specialist Professor Stuart McGill advocates the traditional plank position, my years of experience tell me that it is so often badly executed by non-elite athletes and individuals that the risk-reward ratio for this exercise just doesn't add up.

That said, I agree fully with Professor McGill that variations of the plank like the side plank and Swiss ball plank are essential for engaging and training the core musculature, and my 100,000 system incorporates these essential exercises in all programmes.

Ironically, to achieve the results that you have been promised by performing the plank in the traditional way, you need to completely flip over your body position, as follows. Achieve a much better suspension exercise by following my top tips for this exercise.

- Lie flat on your back.
- Rotate your arms and thumbs outwards (this produces external rotation of your upper arm), then contract and squeeze your shoulder blades together (this produces shoulder girdle retraction, which is beneficial for good posture).
- Lift your hips and pelvis a few inches off the ground and engage your glutes, which are now contracting against a load (gravity) and consequently receiving benefit.

DEVELOPMENT OF MY 100,000 SYSTEM

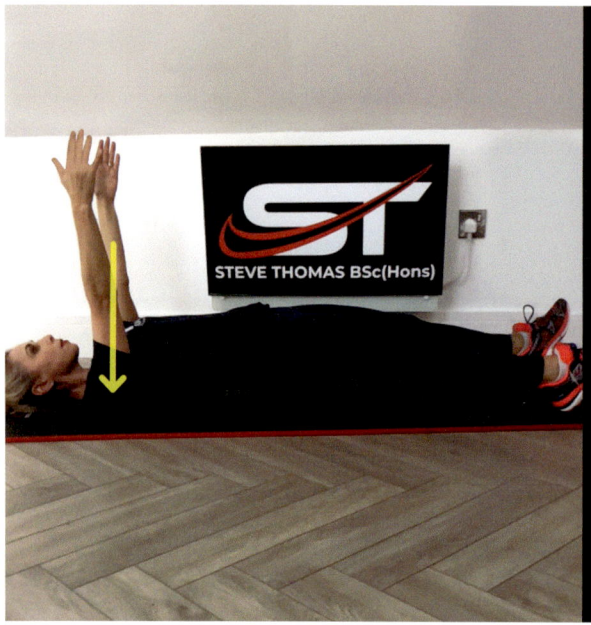

This modified position/technique achieves all the results that you thought were promised from the traditional plank. It increases the strength of the body's posterior chain (the musculature at the rear of the body). Once again, this shows the importance of science, anatomy, biomechanics and detail.

2. Incorrect hamstring stretch

The illustration below depicts a very common way of stretching the hamstring muscles. Indeed, it's universally taught this way. Is this you? Have you been advised to stretch your hamstrings this way? If so, please stop – this is *not* the way to stretch your hamstring muscles.

There is a very simple and yet very important minor modification to this stretching position that you **must** adopt if you want to continue to stretch your hamstrings in this lying position.

Simply reposition your band, rope or towel to cover your heel instead of your forefoot – this allows your foot to relax and, indeed, you should slightly point your toes away from your body (plantar flexion).

This is a much safer and more productive position. The photograph (right) shows how to perform a lying hamstring stretch correctly.

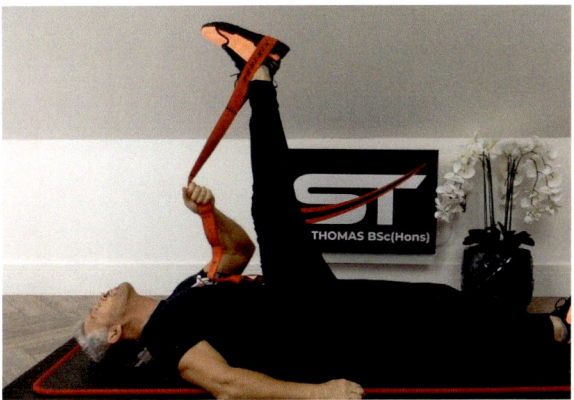

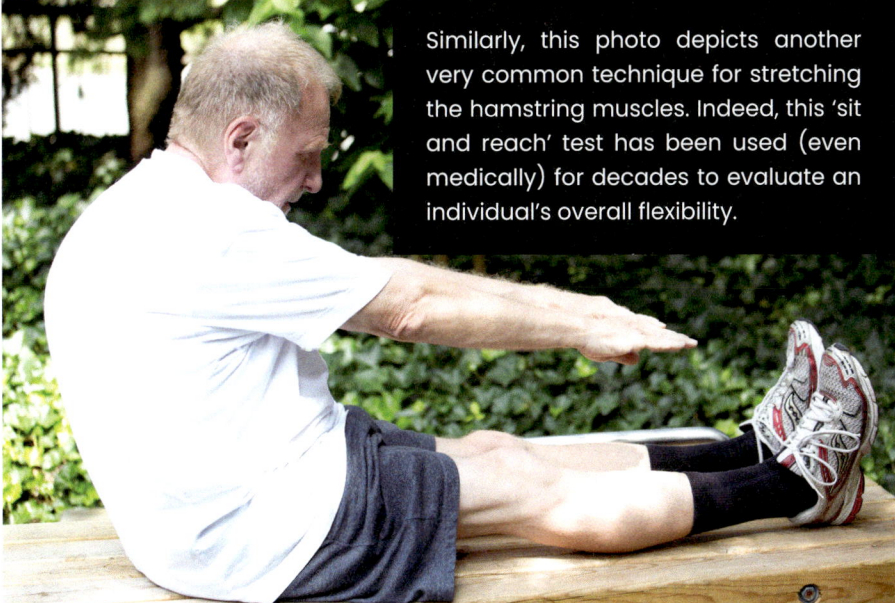

Similarly, this photo depicts another very common technique for stretching the hamstring muscles. Indeed, this 'sit and reach' test has been used (even medically) for decades to evaluate an individual's overall flexibility.

If you have been taught to do it this way, *please stop* – **it is completely wrong**.

In this position:

– The feet are in the **wrong** position (dorsi-flexed).
– The pelvis is at the **wrong** angle (posteriorly tilted).
– The spine is in the **wrong** position (curved/hunched).
– The head and chin are in the **wrong** position (forward and down).
– The arms and hands are in the **wrong** position (pulling the shoulders forward).

DEVELOPMENT OF MY 100,000 SYSTEM

To continue to stretch your hamstrings in this sitting position, you must make critical modifications and adopt the following posture:

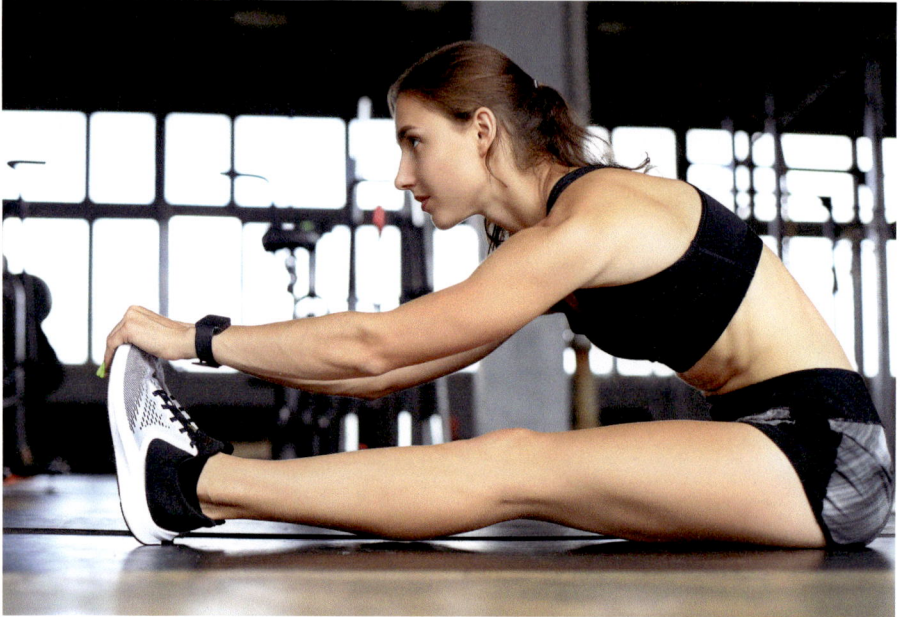

- Point your toes (plantar flexion).
- Anteriorly tilt your pelvis.
- The spine should be in a neutral position.
- The head should be in alignment with the spine (eyes forward).
- The arms and hands should be pointing forward.

Performing your hamstring stretches this way will significantly reduce the tension on both your upper and lower nerve roots and relieve the load on your thoracic (upper) and lumbar (lower) spine. Once again, this is a much safer and more effective stretching position.

Hamstring muscle stretching, both static and dynamic, is a vital component of any exercise routine, but you should never do this stretch with your foot dorsiflexed (toes pointing towards your body). Whether you have been taught this stretch lying down, sitting or standing, and whether you're using a rope, band, towel or just your hands or arms, you should always have your toes and foot in a relaxed position or even plantar-flexed (toes pointing away from your body).

A dorsiflexed foot position can put enormous strain on your body's nerve roots – nerves don't like to be stretched or tensioned – they should glide or slide. Stretching nerves incorrectly can inflame and cause pain, numbness and tingling anywhere along the nerve root.

Irrespective of your body position (lying, sitting, standing), your foot should be relaxed, almost pointed, to release the nerves and ensure that the position does indeed produce a great hamstring muscle stretch. Correct alignment or tilting of the pelvis is crucial, and the spine should be well aligned with the head and neck, not excessively loading the thoracic and lumbar spine.

In conclusion, "the optimal hamstring stretch should only stretch the hamstring muscles, without excessive tension of the sciatic nerve" (theprehabguys.com). Follow my 100,000 programmes for all the best hamstring exercises and stretches.

3. Iliotibial (IT) band rolling

Using a roller to 'treat' the iliotibial band has become a staple exercise for millions of individuals around the world. See photo below.

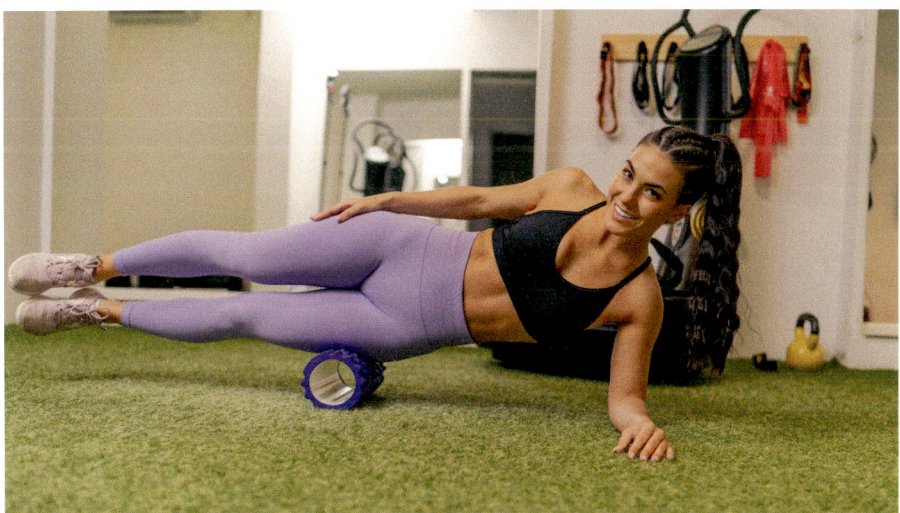

If this is you, stop doing it – stop wasting your time. IT band syndrome (ITBS) is very common and must be treated – but treated correctly.

The sharp, nagging, inflammatory pain caused by ITBS is usually experienced on the outside of the knee. The IT band itself is not a muscle but thick fascia

DEVELOPMENT OF MY 100,000 SYSTEM

(connective tissue), and the pain is usually caused by continual, repetitive friction on the outside of the knee joint, frequently from repetitive actions or activities like running.

Rolling the IT band, if it's inflamed, may inflame it further. Rolling the outer portion of the thigh *muscle*, and more importantly, rolling, stretching and exercising the muscles that attach to the IT band (tensor fascia latae, gluteus medius) constitute the best way, along with massage treatment, to rehabilitate IT band syndrome.

Refer to the 'missing links' section later in this chapter for more information regarding the gluteus medius muscle. The images below show how to roll the TFL (a) and gluteus medius (b).

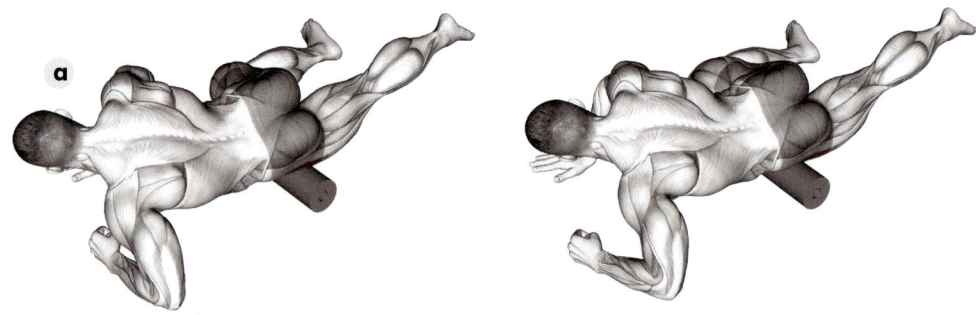

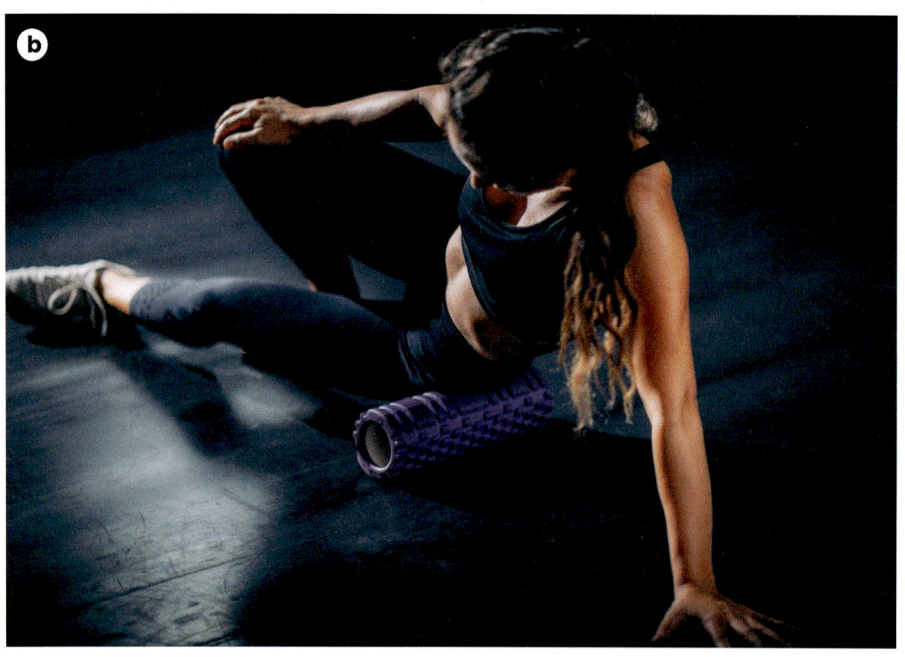

DEVELOPMENT OF MY 100,000 SYSTEM

4. Chest and shoulder exercises (shoulder inflammation)

Almost every past and present exercise, gym routine and weight training programme relies heavily on the following, traditional movements:

a. Chest barbell press
b. Shoulder barbell press
c. Chest dumb-bell fly
d. Lateral shoulder raises
e. Frontal shoulder raises
f. Upright barbell row
g. Press-ups
h. Tricep dips
i. Face pull

If you include any or all these above movements regularly in your gym routines, and more importantly, perform them with standard, traditional technique, **please stop doing them**.

It may sound controversial, but these exercises are not correct and I don't advocate performing them in the normal or traditional way.

All these movements performed repetitively, especially with heavy weights, can put an enormous strain on the shoulder joint. This joint is very complex, with a great range of movement, but the complexity of multidirectional movement patterns leads to vulnerability in certain positions, actions and movements.

Let's consider these movements in more detail.

a. Chest barbell press (shown below)

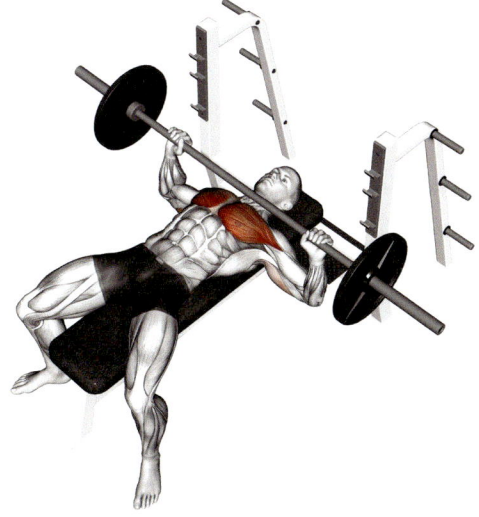 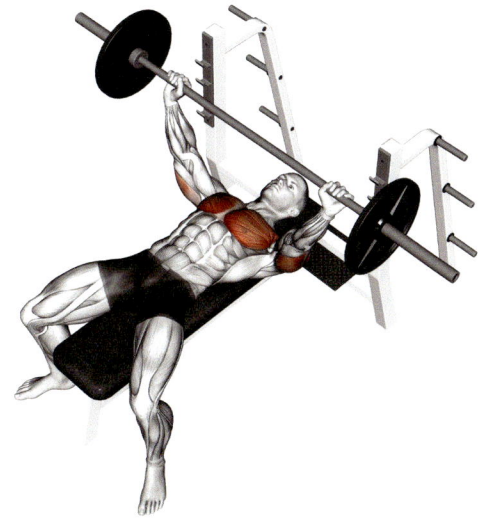

The **FATHER FIGURE** of **FITNESS**

DEVELOPMENT OF MY 100,000 SYSTEM

No gym or weight-training programme ever formulated does not contain this traditional chest exercise – it's almost always the first exercise on the list. The issues I have with the movement are as follows.

First, it is regarded as a strength, mass, bulk-building exercise for the chest, and this alone encourages the belief that it is an essential exercise that should be performed with ever-increasing weight. Technically, at the bottom (starting point) of the chest press, with the elbows out wide to the side, where the joint is at its weakest position, especially with heavy weights, the biomechanical stress on the shoulder joint and capsule is enormous. So we have maximum load at the joint's weakest position. Similarly, at the top (end position) of the movement, when the joint is in its strongest position, the load is at its minimum.

Second, this exercise does not maximise the muscles' capacity for adduction (pulling the arm across the body).

Third, the traditional grip position, with the thumb underneath the bar, encourages slight internal rotation of the upper arm (humerus), which is completely wrong for the shoulder joint.

All these issues add up to a risk/reward ratio that simply doesn't make sense. **It's just not worth it**.

b. Shoulder barbell press

The photo below depicts the standard behind-the-neck (military) shoulder press

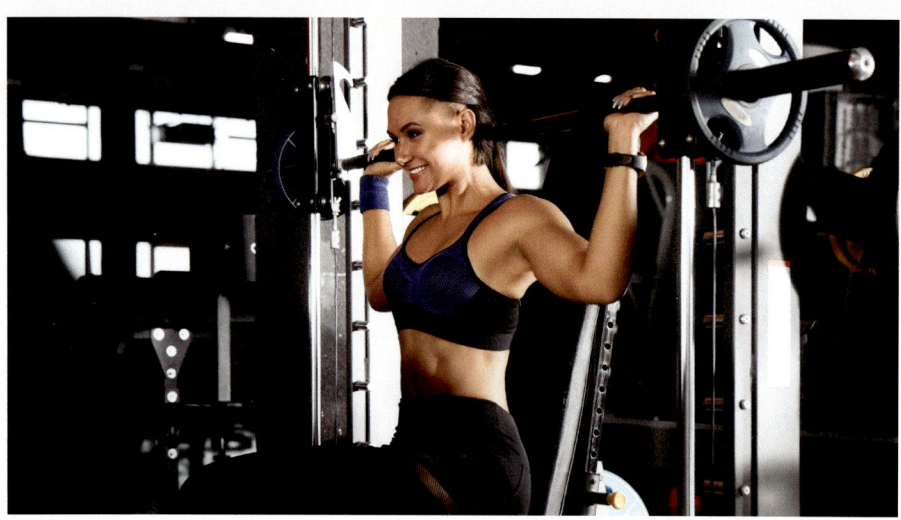

DEVELOPMENT OF MY 100,000 SYSTEM

exercise that has been a staple shoulder exercise for many decades.

This position or technique puts increased loading through the upper back (thoracic) region, neck (cervical) region and the shoulder joint. It simply fights against the human anatomy of the upper back and shoulder, especially with the arms out wide and elbows pushed backward. It is simply nonsensical to try to exercise your shoulders with this technique, especially as there are many safer, more effective alternatives.

c. Chest dumb-bell fly

The below photo depicts the traditional, standard chest dumb-bell fly exercise, another that has been a must-do movement for all chest muscle routines. You have probably been told that this exercise is great because it achieves a much greater stretch across the chest than any other movement.

Analysis of this exercise leads to the same conclusions as those observed with the chest press. The 'great' stretch is precisely why this exercise performed in the traditional way is so bad.

This stretch occurs at the bottom position of the movement, exactly at the point where there is no support for the over-extension of the anterior shoulder capsule.

Please trust me when I say that continued repetitive use of this exercise performed in the traditional way will destroy your shoulder joint capsule.

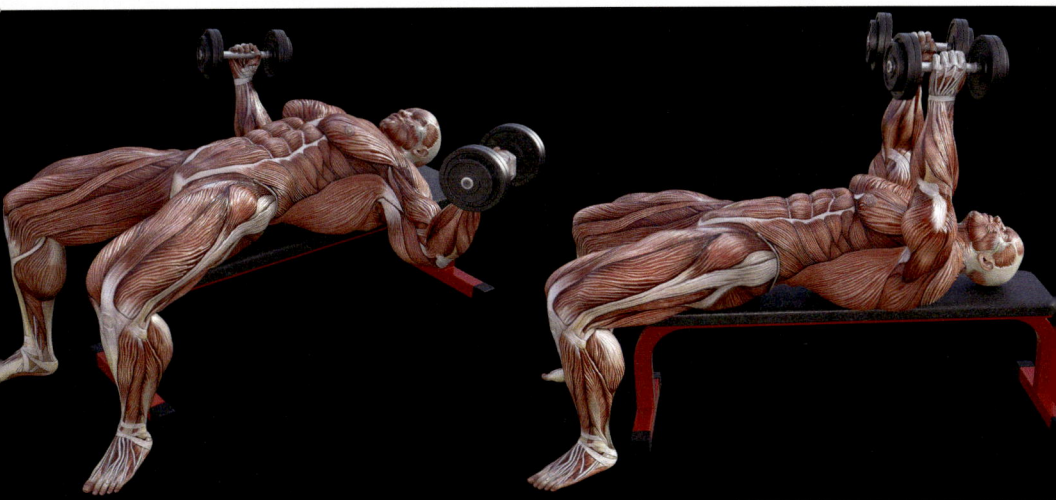

DEVELOPMENT OF MY 100,000 SYSTEM

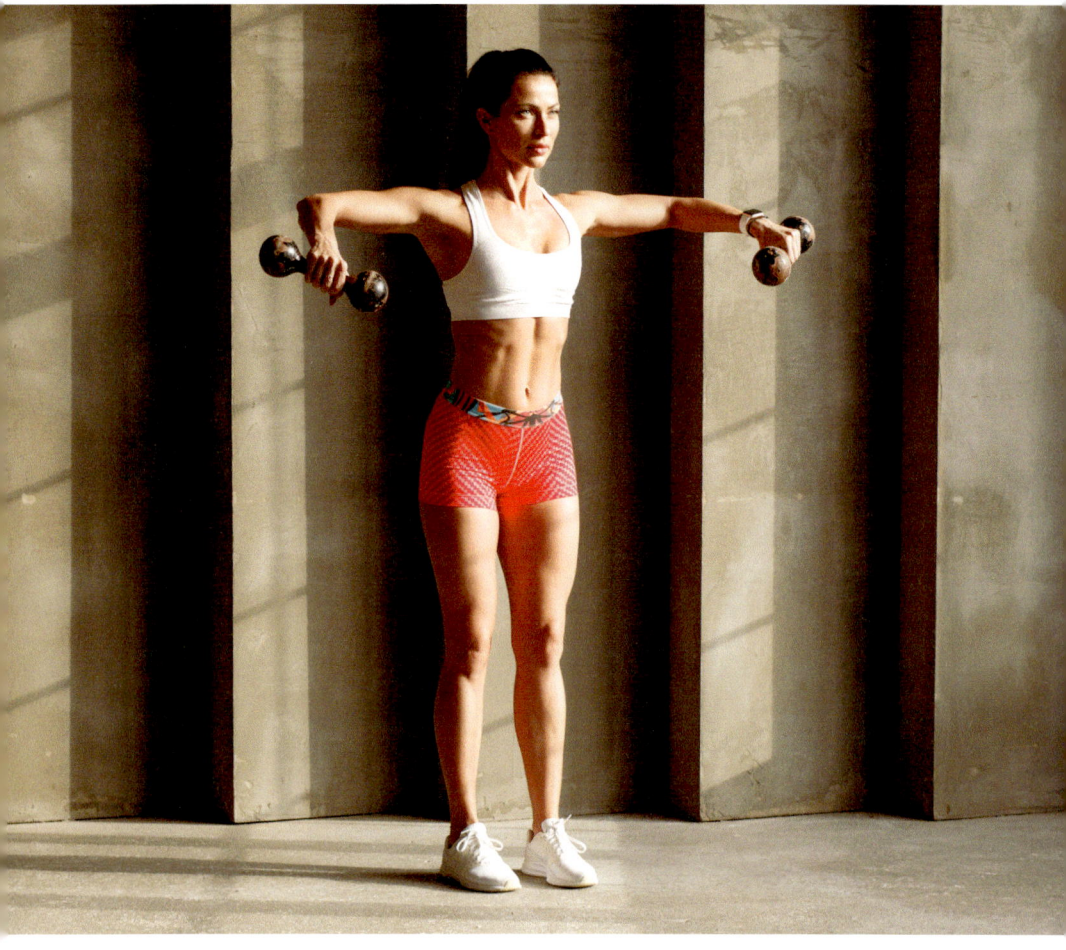

d. Lateral shoulder dumb-bell raise

The photo above depicts the traditional or standard lateral shoulder dumb-bell raise. This exercise performed in the traditional manner has been taught for decades as the best exercise to build and shape the shoulder (deltoid) muscles.

Teachers, coaches and personal trainers frequently encourage individuals to rotate the thumbs downward as the individual lifts the weight up to the side. This variation, in particular, is very bad – the downward thumb rotation causes excess internal rotation of the upper arm (humerus), loading the rotator cuff, and combining this with the elevation of the upper arm makes it a lethal combination for the rotator cuff and shoulder joint. You simply **must not** perform it this way.

DEVELOPMENT OF MY 100,000 SYSTEM

e. Frontal shoulder dumb-bell raises

The illustration (right) depicts the frontal shoulder dumb-bell raise exercise, which has been used for decades to strengthen, build and shape the frontal shoulder (anterior deltoid).

The palms-down position employed in this technique again encourages internal rotation of the upper arm (humerus). This internally rotated position puts unnecessary stress and strain on the anterior shoulder capsule and therefore should **never** be executed this way.

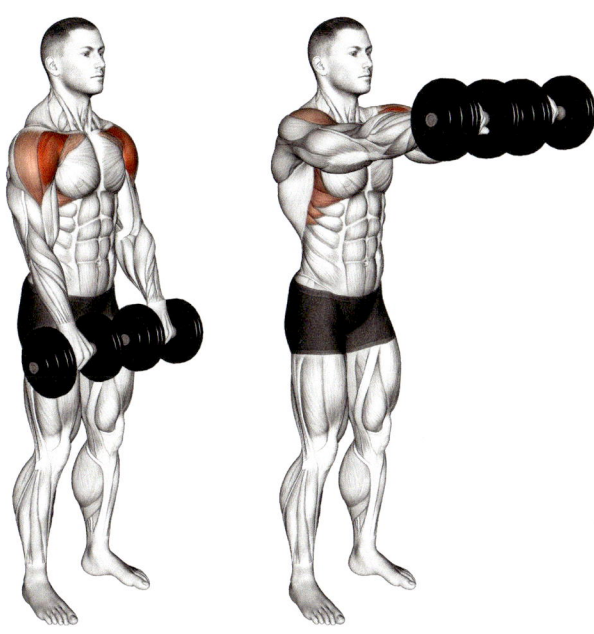

f. Upright barbell/pulley row

Below is an illustration that depicts the traditional or standard upright barbell/pulley row.

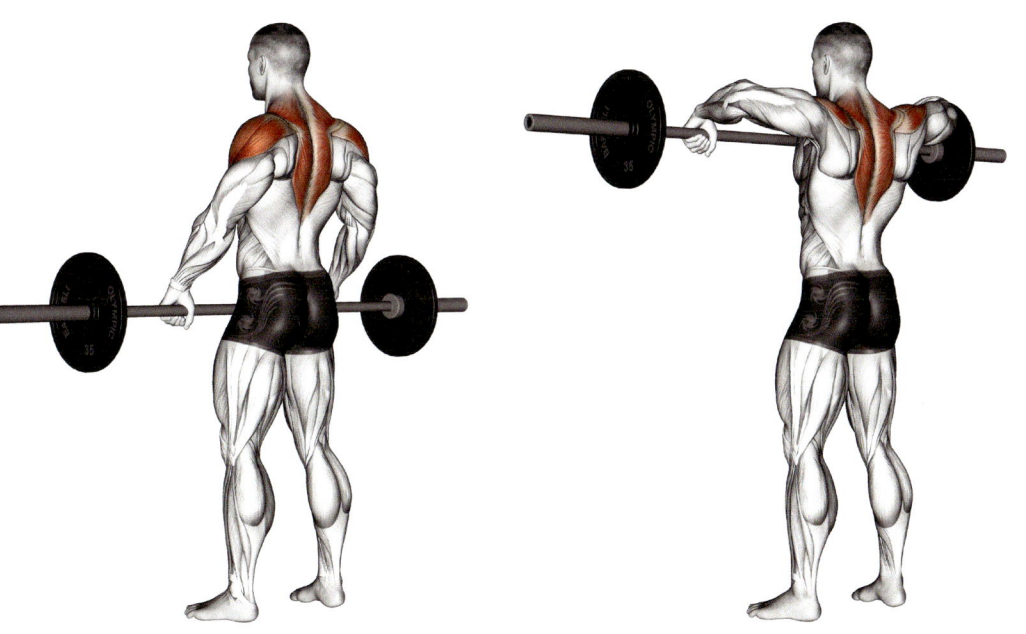

DEVELOPMENT OF MY 100,000 SYSTEM

I fully understand that many top bodybuilders and strength athletes, including legends of the sports, actively endorse this movement as a wonderful frontal shoulder (anterior deltoid) and upper back/neck (trapezius) exercise, but my experience tells me that you should **simply never perform this exercise**.

If there is one position, one movement that hammers the shoulder joint, it's this one. Please forget that this exercise even exists – blank it out completely.

g. Press-up

The illustration below depicts a standard or traditional press-up exercise – a movement that is probably more synonymous with exercising than any other. It has been suggestive of strength and physical power for decades and is often a party piece for anyone 'showing off' his/her upper-body prowess.

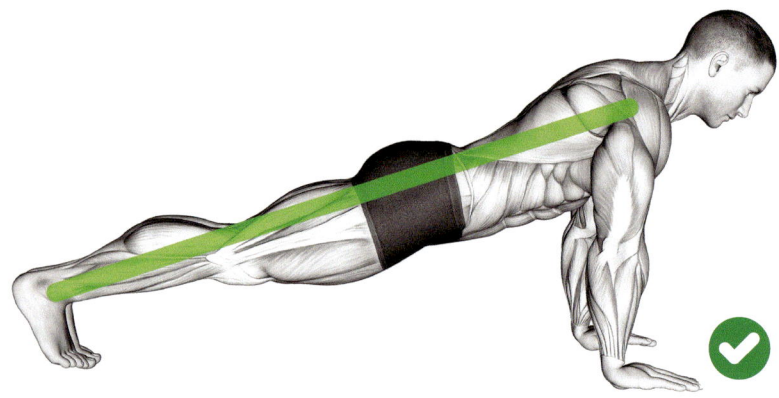

With this press-up movement the correct body position is imperative, but still, to this day, it is often performed incorrectly. In fact, it is probably the most mis-performed exercise of all.

The illustrations below show the common mistakes made: misalignment of the

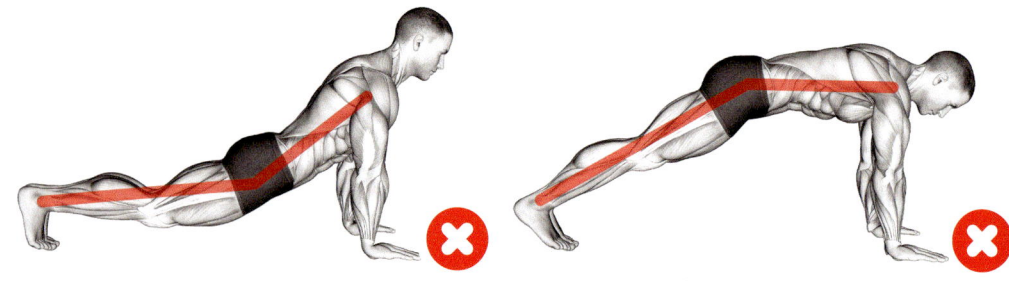

head and neck, shrugging of the shoulders, upper-back curvature, weakness in the lower back and glutes, elbows too wide and high and incorrect position of the hands. All of these errors load the spine incorrectly and put the shoulder girdle, neck, head and shoulder joint in compromised positions, which leads to soreness and pain.

In addition, most individuals 'bounce' through their press-up movements, increasing the load through the joints.

h. Tricep dip

This illustration depicts a standard or traditional tricep dip. This is another exercise that has been regarded as a must-do chest and tricep exercise for decades. I am here to tell you simply to **stop** doing this exercise this way.

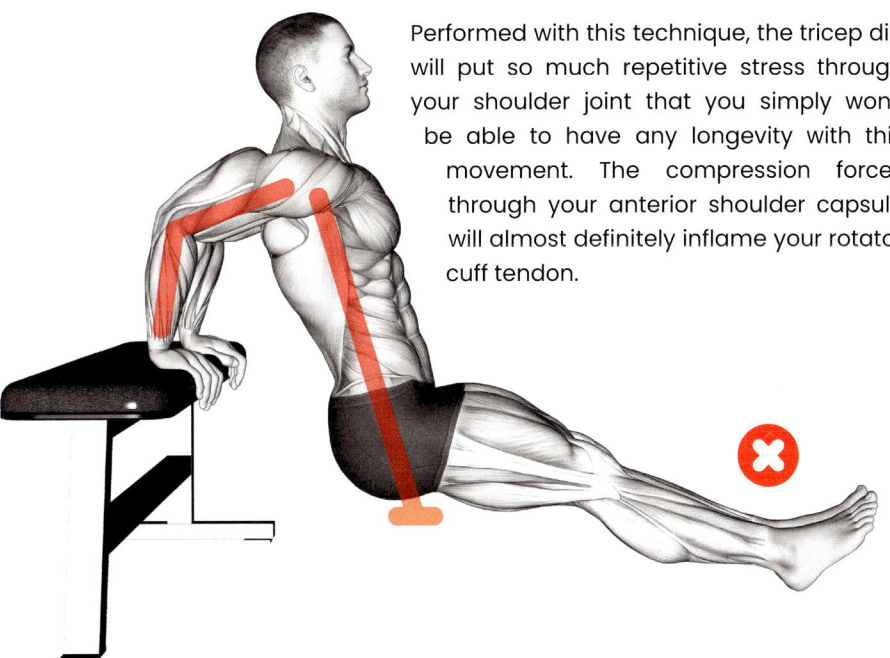

Performed with this technique, the tricep dip will put so much repetitive stress through your shoulder joint that you simply won't be able to have any longevity with this movement. The compression forces through your anterior shoulder capsule will almost definitely inflame your rotator cuff tendon.

I believe that this exercise performed with this technique is a disaster for your shoulder joints, so please learn from my experience and **never** perform it this way, especially as there is a very simple alternative.

i. Face pull

This illustration depicts a standard or traditional face pull pulley exercise, a much more recent addition to the exercise 'pool'. It has become popular, but this technique is **completely wrong**.

The intended purpose of this movement is to perform shoulder retraction, which should generally be encouraged – it's necessary for good thoracic, head and neck posture. I stated above that the upright rowing movement is the worst possible exercise for your shoulder joints, and close inspection of the traditional face pull shows that the movement is very close to an upright row.

Scientific understanding of your arm and shoulder position and function tells me that this technique simply fights against your own anatomy, putting unnecessary stress through your shoulder joint. Pulling from low to high produces internal rotation with elevation of the upper arm (humerus), which damages the shoulder.

Again, technical modifications are critical for this movement.

As a sport scientist, I understand the functional complexity of shoulder mechanics. These exercises can ravage the shoulder joint like no other exercises, positions or movements. The scientific research literature is in complete agreement, and my experience has shown me first-hand that continued or repetitive use of these exercises performed in the traditional way can lead to inflammation known as shoulder impingement syndrome (SIS) or rotator cuff tendonitis.

SIS is very prevalent in weight trainers, sportsmen and women, gymnasts, all racket sports and athletes, and is often called 'swimmer's shoulder'. It results from continued rubbing of the rotator cuff between the humerus (upper arm bone) and the top outer portion of the shoulder joint. The rubbing leads to swelling and further narrowing of the joint space, resulting in irritation and pain.

It is the cause of up to 65 per cent of all shoulder pain and if left untreated, shoulder impingement syndrome may need anti-inflammatory medication, ice, cortisone injections or surgery.

The above actions, positions, movements, and exercises have another common element that increases the load on the shoulder joint.

During traditional chest muscle exercises, many traditional shoulder exercises and some traditional tricep exercises, the humerus (upper arm) is **internally rotated**. This internally rotated position is a major contributing factor that causes SIS.

External rotation of the arm (humerus), by contrast, affords a greater spacing (gap) in the shoulder joint, for more freedom and more fluid and unhindered shoulder function.

The photograph below shows a clear difference in the orientation of the head of the humerus in the shoulder socket during external rotation.

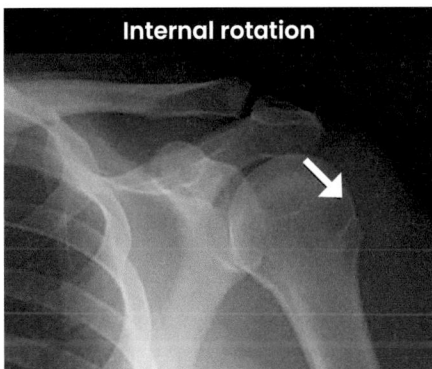
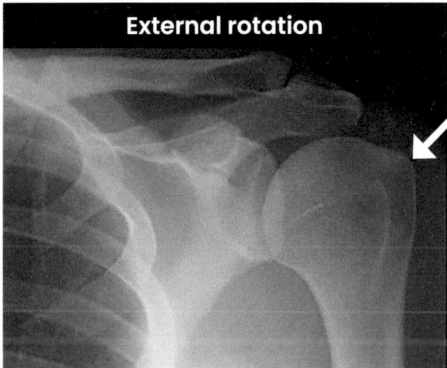

Please remember that **detail matters**, and it is the details of these movements, not necessarily the movements themselves, that are wrong. It is stupid to put unnecessary stress and strain through your vulnerable shoulder joint, when small, easy modifications could save it from inflammation, pain and serious injury. You only have two shoulder joints – *you must look after them*.

Small technical modifications can change the same fundamental movement from a shoulder disaster to a shoulder 'master blaster'.

It is imperative, therefore, to ensure that all of the above exercises for the chest, shoulders, neck, upper back, biceps and triceps are performed with as much **external rotation** of the upper arm (humerus) as possible. This is a non-negotiable, essential rule to safeguard your shoulder joints.

DEVELOPMENT OF MY 100,000 SYSTEM

My 100,000 system incorporates specially modified exercises that reduce the internal rotational stress on the shoulder joint, increasing external rotation, allowing it to perform fluidly and efficiently.

My top tips for the necessary modifications of all the above exercises, to produce greater upper-arm external rotation and significantly reduce unnecessary strain on your shoulder joints, are as follows.

The barbell chest press

If you are hell-bent on doing the barbell chest press, then you **must** adhere to the following four modifications:

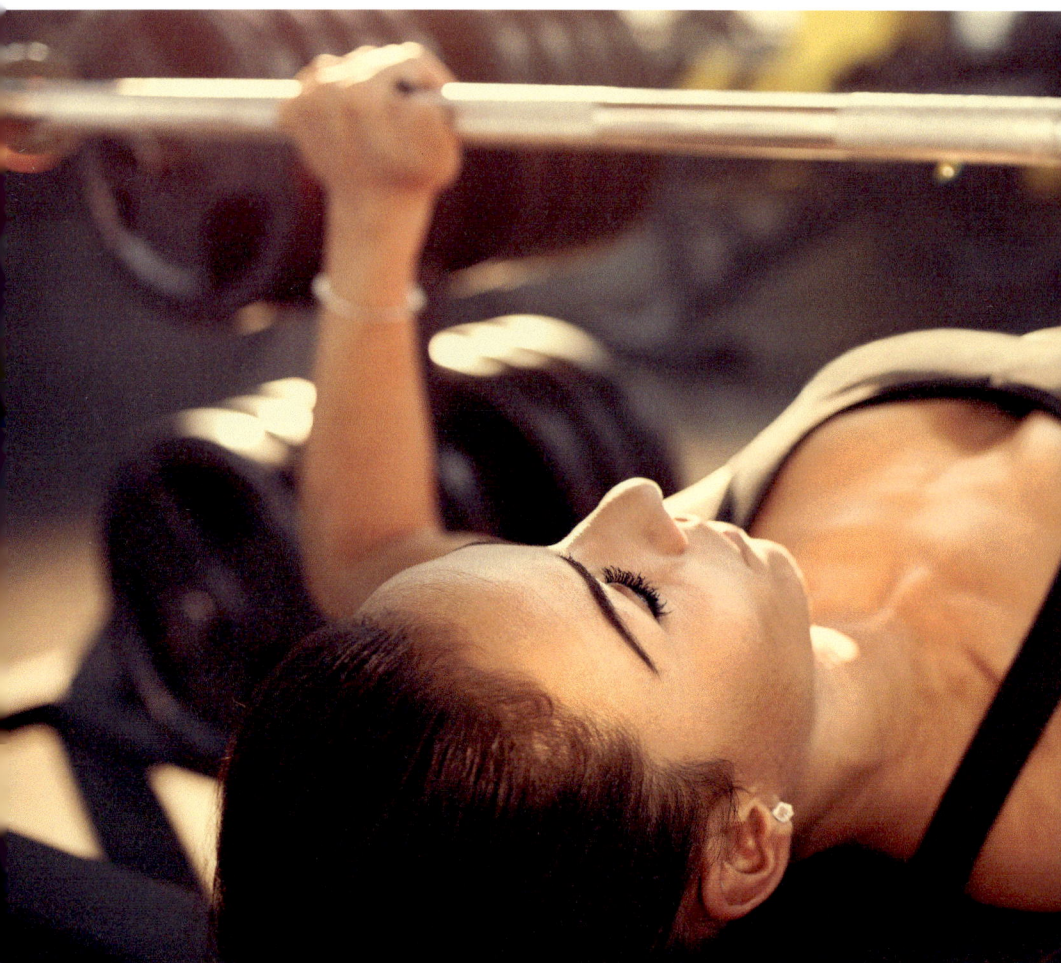

DEVELOPMENT OF MY 100,000 SYSTEM

1. Don't lift super-heavy weights – medium weights only.
2. Don't lower the barbell to full stretching position (reducing the load through the shoulder joint).
3. Don't force your elbows out wide (drop your elbows 30 degrees closer to your side).
4. Change your grip (place your thumb behind the barbell alongside your fingers), as shown in Photo (right).

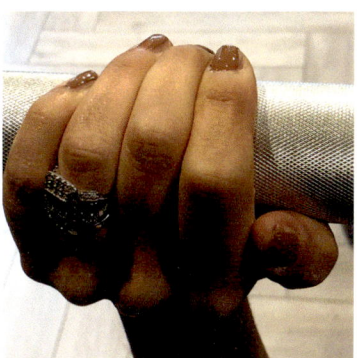

The following photograph shows how to perform a barbell chest press correctly.

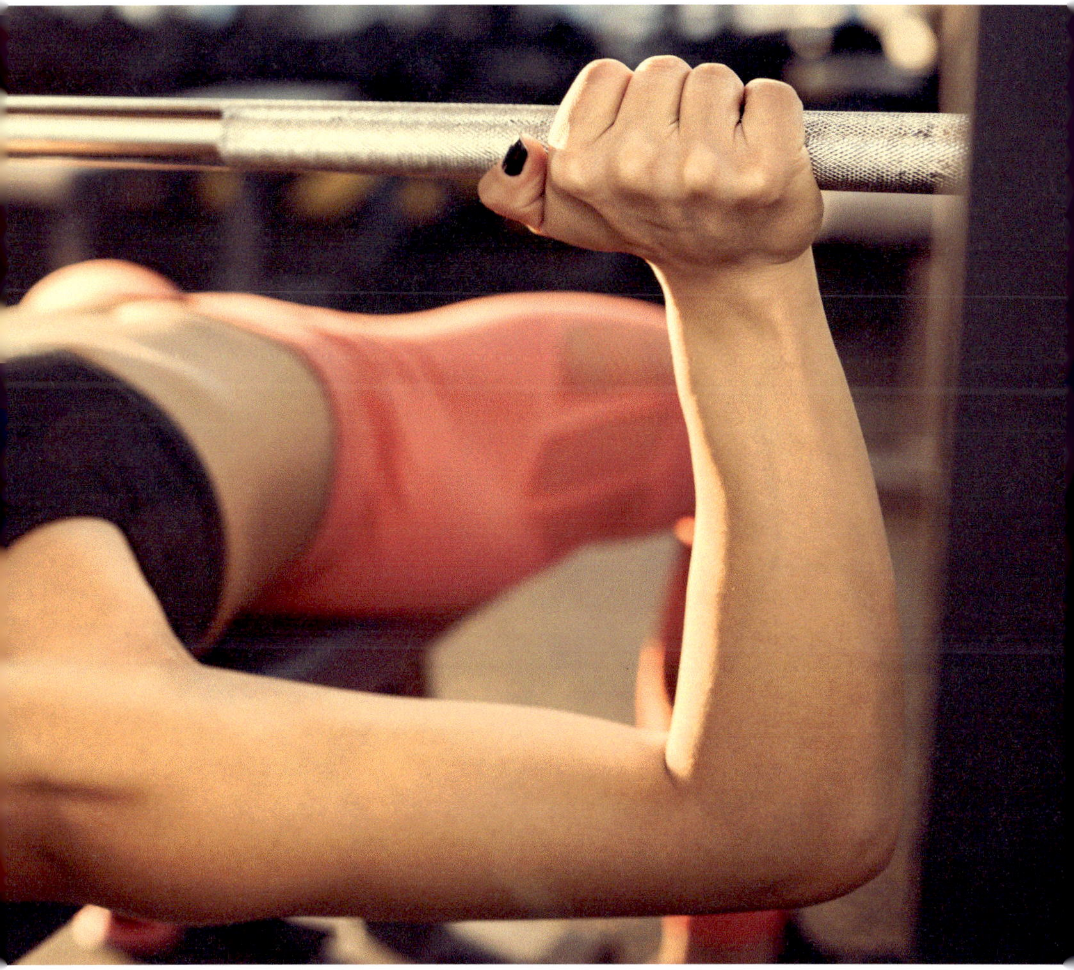

DEVELOPMENT OF MY 100,000 SYSTEM

Shoulder barbell press

The decisive factor again is within the detail. Small, simple modifications can transform this posture and shoulder 'crunching' exercise into a very safe, efficient and productive movement, taking great load away from the joint and isolating the shoulder (deltoid) musculature.

Overhead barbell shoulder press **must** be performed with the following technique.

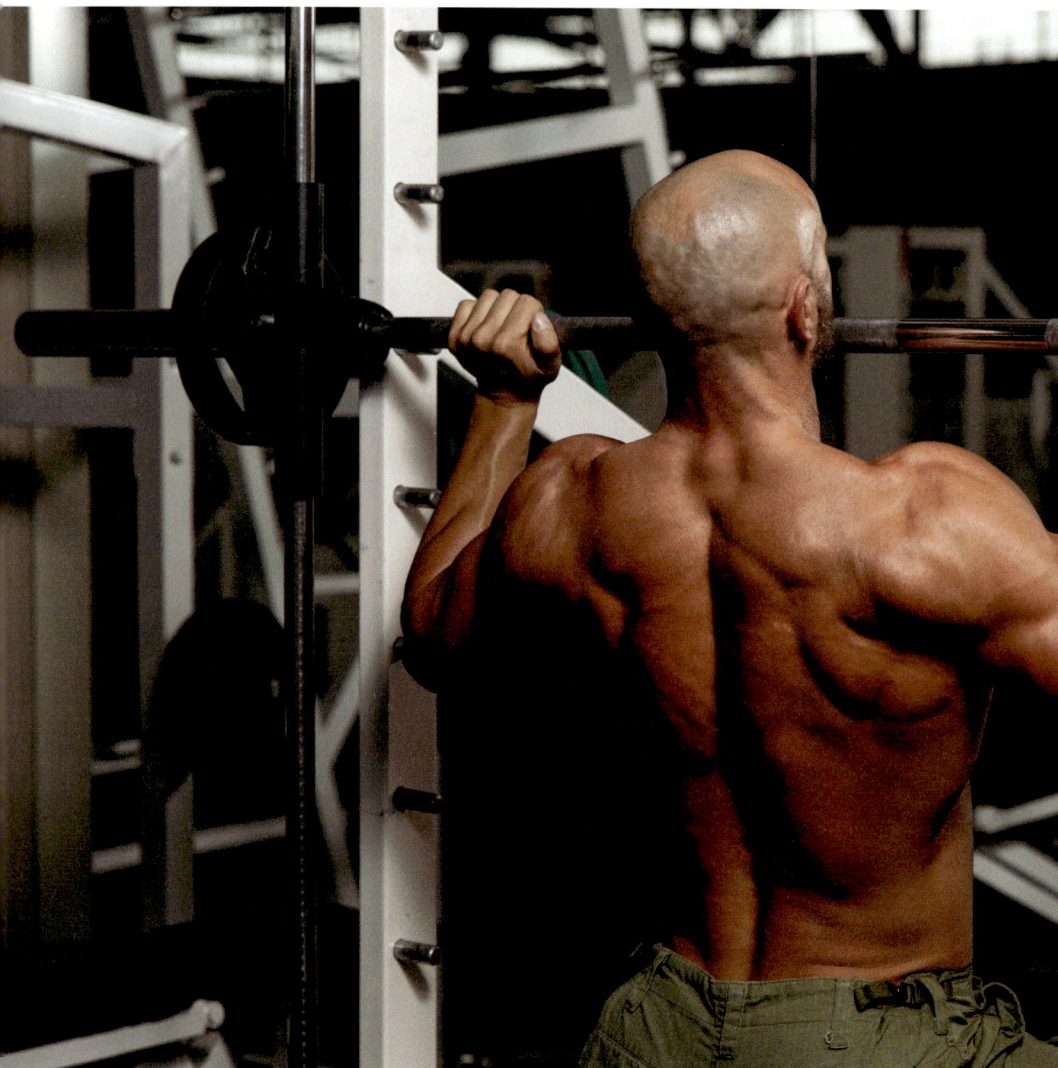

DEVELOPMENT OF MY 100,000 SYSTEM

1. The barbell must be in front of the head (reducing the shoulder girdle and postural load).
2. Retract/stabilise the shoulder girdle (this helps maintain good posture of the thoracic spine).
3. Don't lift super-heavy weight (medium weight only).
4. Keep your elbows slightly down and forward (reduces shoulder joint strain).
5. Change your grip (as above, this encourages slight external rotation of the arm).

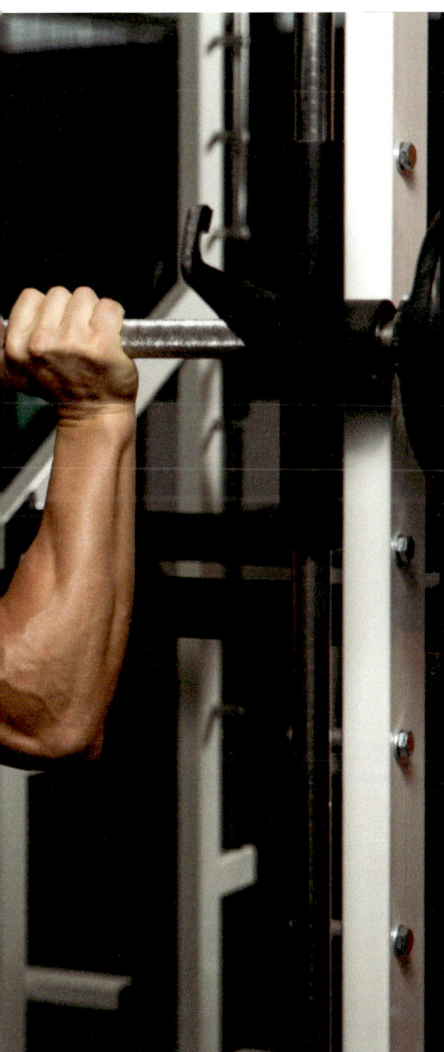

Both of the above exercises, the barbell chest press and the barbell shoulder press, are standard exercises that millions of individuals around the world are performing as you read this book. My **top tips** for modifying these exercises are very simple, and the change of grip position is another **golden rule** to adhere to.

These barbell exercises should be 'pushed' vertically and so it's quite simple to 'cup' the bar with your hands, removing your thumb from underneath the bar, relaxing your grip and pulling your thumb back behind the bar to align with your fingers. This slight change will minimise internal rotation of your upper arm (humerus) in the shoulder joint.

These combined modifications encourage slightly greater external rotation of your upper arm (humerus) and give a much better arm angle which, in turn, reduces the load through your joint. This will give you long-term management of your vulnerable shoulder, and it may just save your gym, weight-training or sporting career.

DEVELOPMENT OF MY 100,000 SYSTEM

Chest dumb-bell fly

To continue using this chest movement in your routines, you **must** adhere to the following technique modifications. They will take substantial load off your shoulder joint, allowing for greater biomechanical protection.

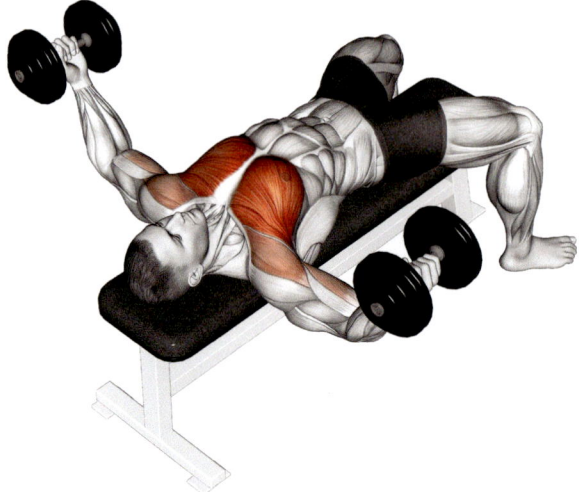

1. Do *not* use maximum weight (light or medium weights only).
2. Bend your elbows (never perform with straight elbow joints).
3. Keep your elbows/arms 30 degrees closer to your side (reduces shoulder joint strain).
4. Externally rotate your arms and weights 45 degrees (lead the movement with the little fingers).

These simple changes not only produce a safer externally rotated position of the arm, they also allow for greater adduction (pulling the arm further across the chest, to the breast bone) and a greater 'squeeze' across the chest (a greater range of movement),

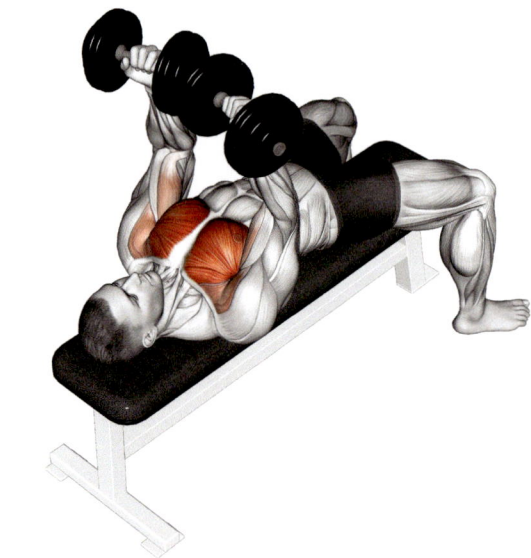

making this movement safer and more productive. This modification should become the normal way of performing and teaching this exercise.

DEVELOPMENT OF MY 100,000 SYSTEM

Lateral shoulder dumb-bell raise

With a few simple modifications that will take a significant load away from the shoulder joint, we can turn this 'lethal' shoulder exercise into a safe and effective version.

1. Do *not* use maximum weight (light or medium weights only).
2. Bend your elbows (never perform with straight elbow joints).
3. Rotate the weights 90 degrees upwards (aids external rotation of the upper arms).
4. Rotate your hands/arms 90 degrees upwards (produces external rotation of the upper arm).
5. Point your thumbs upwards (towards the ceiling).

These simple changes not only produce a much safer externally rotated position of the upper arm, they also allow for a greater range of movement and greater abduction (lifting the arm up and away from the midline of the body), making the modification far superior to the traditional movement. Again, this **must** become the normal way of performing or teaching this exercise.

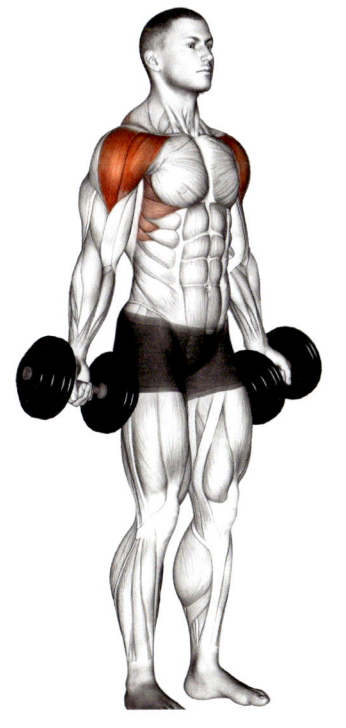
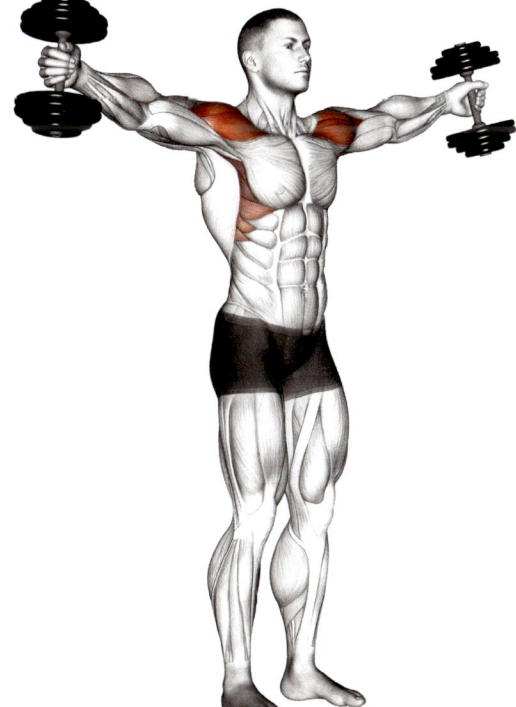

DEVELOPMENT OF MY 100,000 SYSTEM

Frontal shoulder dumb-bell raise

We can turn this destructive shoulder exercise into a much better, safer and more efficient shoulder (deltoid) exercise, by following the above advice for the lateral raise:

1. Do *not* use maximum weight (light or medium weights only).
2. Slightly bend your elbows (your arms should not be rigid).
3. Rotate the dumb-bells 90 degrees upwards (aids external rotation of the upper arm).
4. Rotate your hands/arms 90 degrees upwards (produces external rotation of the upper arm).
5. Point the thumbs upwards (towards the ceiling).

These simple changes produce a much safer externally rotated position of the upper arm and allow for a greater range of movement (arm flexion), making this variation a far superior movement to the traditional one. Once again, this **must** become the normal way of performing and teaching this exercise.

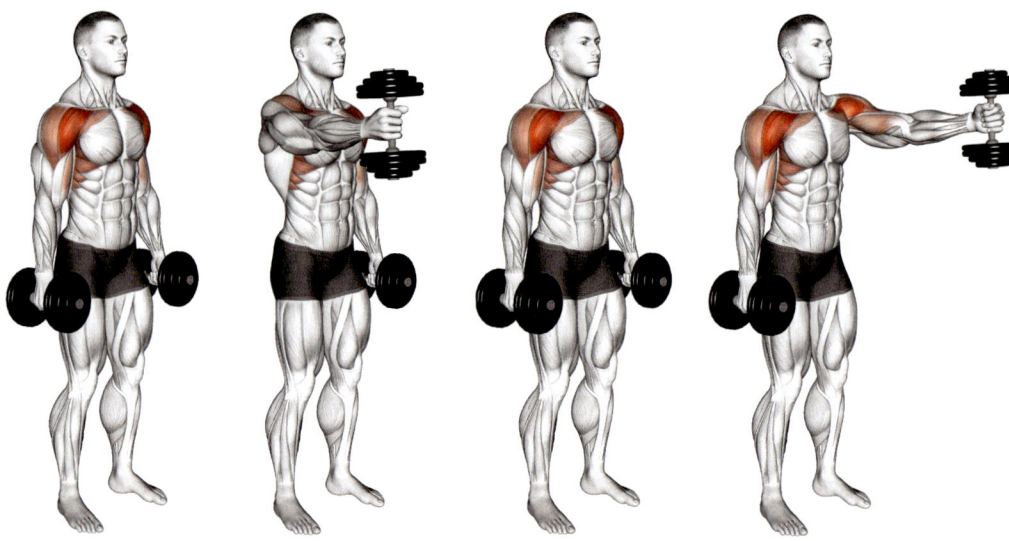

Press-up

The main issue with press-ups is that almost everyone cheats, intentionally or unintentionally, at every possible opportunity. As I've already said, it's probably the most incorrectly performed exercise of all.

The fundamental reason why a press-up is such a staple of every exercise routine is clear – functional body weight movements have certainly earned the right to be appreciated and included in most exercise routines.

The key, again, is in the detail. It is imperative that the body positions are correct and that individuals truly understand what they are doing, and why.

To turn a mis-performed, hence destructive, exercise for your back, neck and shoulders, into a good, safe and more productive chest and shoulder exercise, you **must** perform them correctly. The following modifications must be adhered to:

1. Head/neck position (this must maintain a neutral position).
2. Shoulder position (important not to shrug the shoulders – consciously 'un-shrug' them).
3. Upper back position (create stability by pulling the shoulder blades back and down).
4. Activate the gluteal muscles (contract the glutes to help fix the position of the mid/upper back and shoulder girdle).
5. Elbow position (don't let the elbows travel high; bring them 30 degrees down into the side of the body).
6. Angle of push (don't push vertically but slightly backwards).
7. Tempo of the movement (*no* bouncing, *no* momentum, pause at the top and bottom).
8. Hand position (turn the hands 30-40 degrees outwards, promoting external arm rotation).

These simple changes produce a much safer externally rotated position of the upper arm and maintain the position, posture and biomechanical integrity of the entire body, making it a far superior method to the traditional technique.

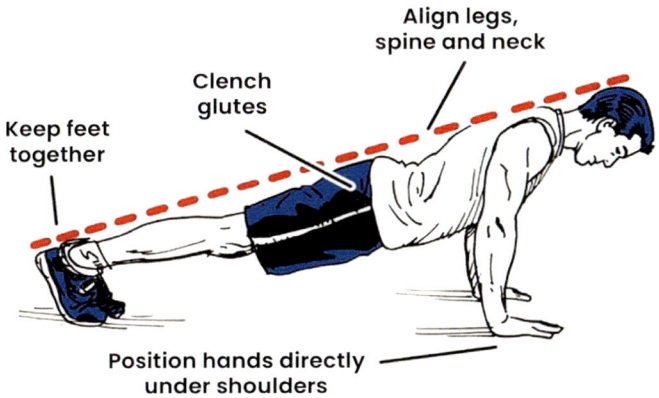

DEVELOPMENT OF MY 100,000 SYSTEM

Tricep dip

As we've seen, the traditional tricep dip technique encourages bad posture and bad shoulder girdle position, and the resulting hunching of the spine creates havoc in the shoulder. If you are to perform this movement correctly and productively, the following modifications **must** be adhered to:

1. You must retract your shoulders (pull the shoulder girdles back and down to ensure shoulder joint and shoulder girdle stability and good posture).
2. Rotate the hand grip position outwards 70-90 degrees (producing external rotation).

These simple modifications will change this exercise from being a **disaster** for your shoulders into a safe, strong and productive movement for your chest and shoulder muscles.

The face pull

The traditional technique for the face pull is another disaster for the shoulder. This is, however, an important exercise that we should all be encouraged to perform more regularly. The movement performed correctly is beneficial to posture, stability and health.

Even though there are numerous tutorials promoting bad technique, please trust me to show you how to perform this exercise properly. The key elements are, height, stance, grip and movement.

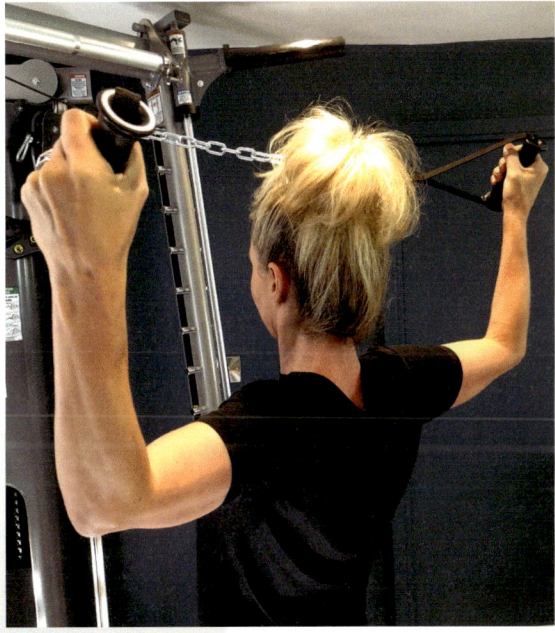

1. Do *not* pull from low to high. This encourages bad posture, pulling the upper body forward and down.
2. Pull from high to lower. This produces the desired angle to engage the rear shoulders (deltoids), the rhomboids and trapezius (upper back).
3. Adopt a square stance. This helps to regulate the weight.
4. Change the overhand grip to an underhand grip (point the thumbs upwards to ensure external rotation of the upper arm).
5. The movement should pull to the face, with the hands being pulled backwards further than the elbows. This produces external rotation, opens up the chest, allows a squeeze through the back and exercises the rotator cuff.

These are critical modifications that change the worst possible exercise into one of the best. This modified exercise can now be used regularly and repeatedly to rectify the modern-day phenomenon of bad postural habits leading to 'tech neck'.

5. Squat

The squat exercise has been a staple of almost every exercise programme for decades with a reputation of being a must-do for anyone who is serious about their health and fitness. Essentially, it is a good movement, productive and efficient, and it's important to include squats in your routines, but **only** if you can perform them correctly.

I'm sure you have heard or been taught that you must engage your core, get into a deep knee-bent position, keep your back flat and never let your knees go in front of your toes. The variations in technique that I have observed over many decades while individuals try to adhere to these instructions are staggering. The illustration (right) shows a technique that is **completely wrong**.

From a scientific viewpoint, the above advice is nothing short of nonsense. What exactly does it even mean?

The human spine is curved (S-shaped). It never has been flat, never will be flat, and what's more, should never be flat.

An individual's ability to perform the squat movement properly depends on many anatomical and biomechanical factors:

- ankle joint mobility
- hip anatomical restrictions
- hip capsular mobility
- pelvic stability
- pelvic muscle tightness.
  Biomechanically speaking, good squatting technique requires:
- the head to be upright
- the spine to be in the 'neutral' position
- the abdominals and gluteals to be engaged
- the hips and the chest to move together to provide stability and engage the core muscles

– the knees to be slightly in front of the toes
– the bar or dumb-bells to move vertically.

Furthermore, as I have shown, only a small percentage of individuals have good body mechanics, so squatting is simply not for everyone. Due to the technical difficulties and biomechanical issues presented by the squat, I do not advocate deep knee bending, especially with heavy weights.

As I described in Chapter 7, foot pronation and knee valgum are common mechanical issues, and squatting will expose and exacerbate these issues, producing bad movements with potential for pain and injury.

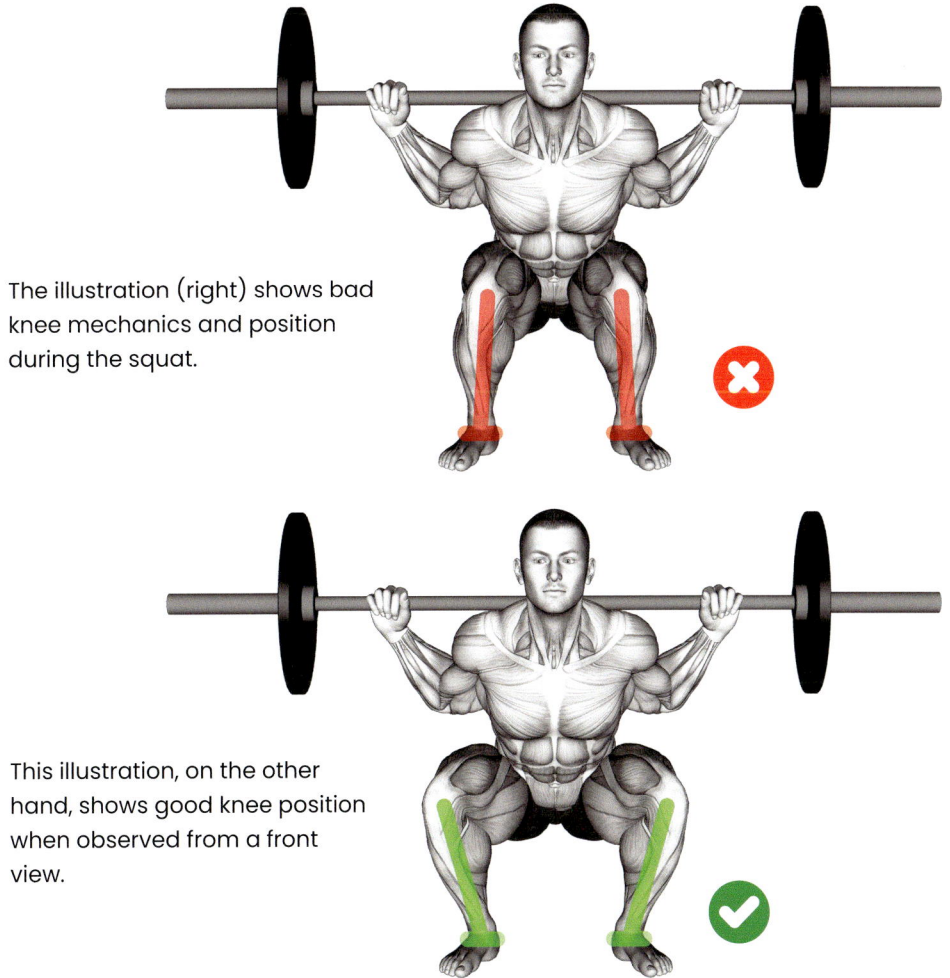

The illustration (right) shows bad knee mechanics and position during the squat.

This illustration, on the other hand, shows good knee position when observed from a front view.

DEVELOPMENT OF MY 100,000 SYSTEM

This common mechanical issue also highlights the lack of strength and inefficiency of the gluteal muscles, specifically the gluteus medius.

To address and rectify this inefficient movement, I advocate that all squatting movements should be performed with an elastic band, positioned just above the knee joints, to provide the necessary resistance to activate, engage and hence exercise the gluteus medius during squatting movements. The photograph (right) represents this modified squatting movement.

This modified technique not only activates and engages the gluteus medius, making it a far superior squatting movement mechanically, it also encourages the individual to perform slower, more considered repetitions, ensuring greater consideration of foot, ankle, knee, hip, pelvis, spine, neck and head position.

My 100,000 system incorporates only specially modified squatting exercises, to ensure results while aiding body posture, mechanics, back and knee function.

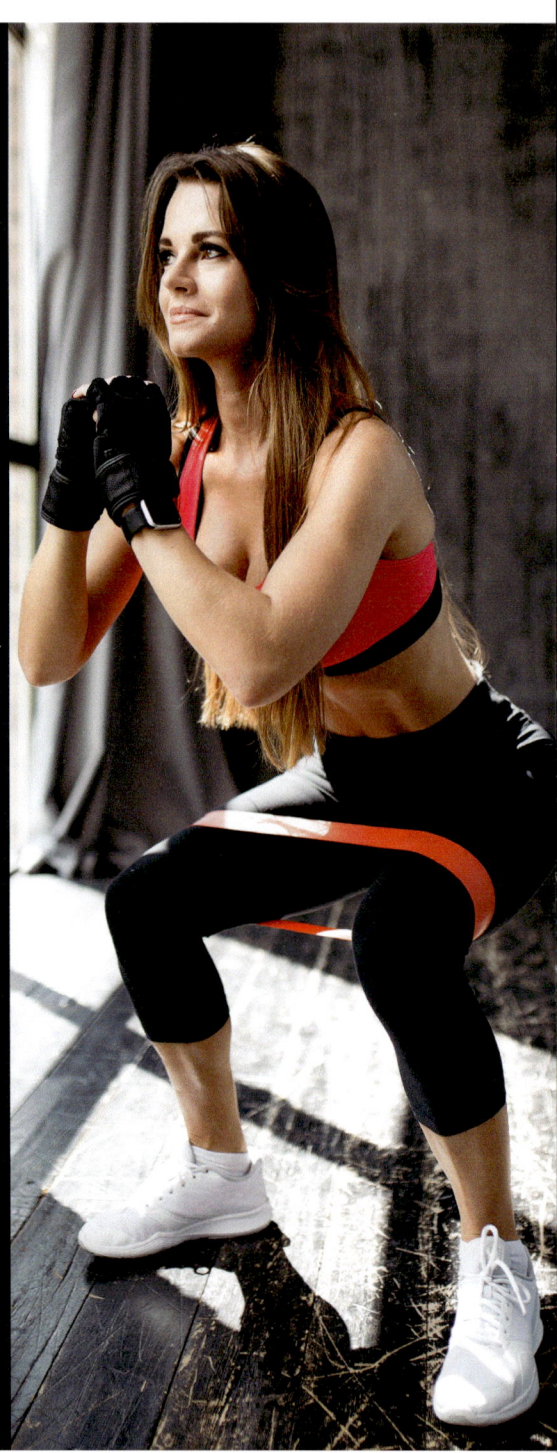

DEVELOPMENT OF MY 100,000 SYSTEM

6. Leg extension machine

The leg extension machine exercise, as seen in the illustration below, is another that has been a staple of almost all exercise and gym routines for decades.

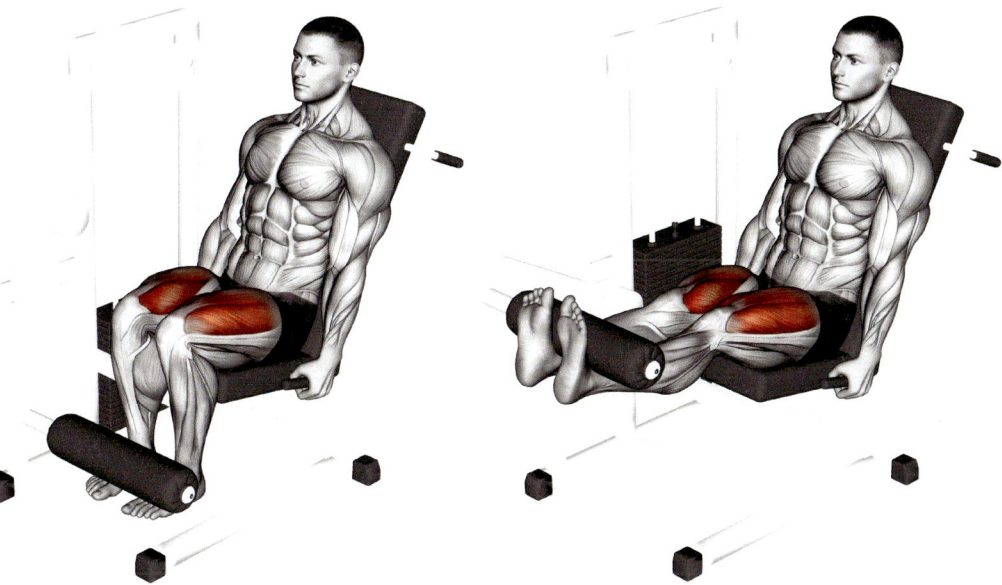

Growing scientific understanding of body mechanics and knee function suggests caution with this exercise. With full range of movement there exists a 'dislocation force' that simply cannot be ignored, especially while using heavy resistance or weights.

I advocate a modified version of this machine exercise, with **very light** resistance and over a very **small range of movement** (the end range of ten to 15 degrees), to isolate the inner portion of the thigh/quadriceps muscle (vastus medialis). The photograph (right) depicts this modified movement.

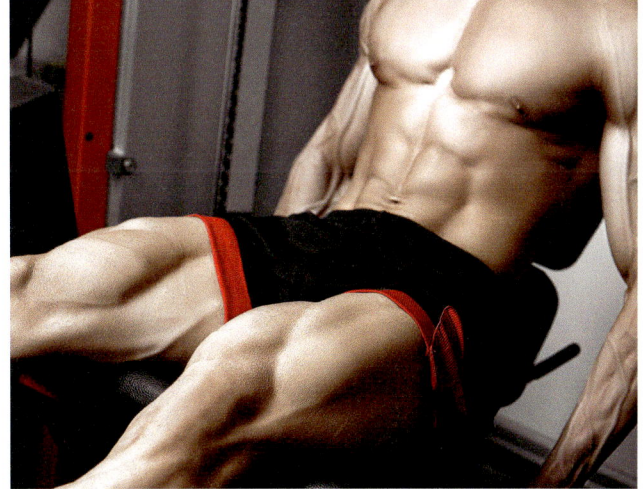

The FATHER FIGURE of FITNESS

DEVELOPMENT OF MY 100,000 SYSTEM

This modified, short-range version of the leg extension is essential for the position and movement of the kneecap (patella) and vital for knee function and health. Learn from my knowledge and experience: stay away from potentially problematic movements, only incorporating my specially modified movements.

7. Behind-the-neck pulldown (lat pulldown)

This is an out-of-date exercise and simply **wrong**. Please, please **stop** using it!

I have already discussed the modern-day pandemic of 'tech neck', how destructive it can be to one's posture and the increased loading it puts through the upper back, neck and shoulder joints and musculature. It's simply nonsensical to continue to use this movement.

The fact that many famous bodybuilders built impressive upper-body musculature utilising this movement for decades is simply not a good reason to continue its use, especially as the identical lat pulldown movement, with the bar in front of the head, is a far superior movement that produces equal results and also reduces excess stress and strain on the vulnerable shoulder joint.

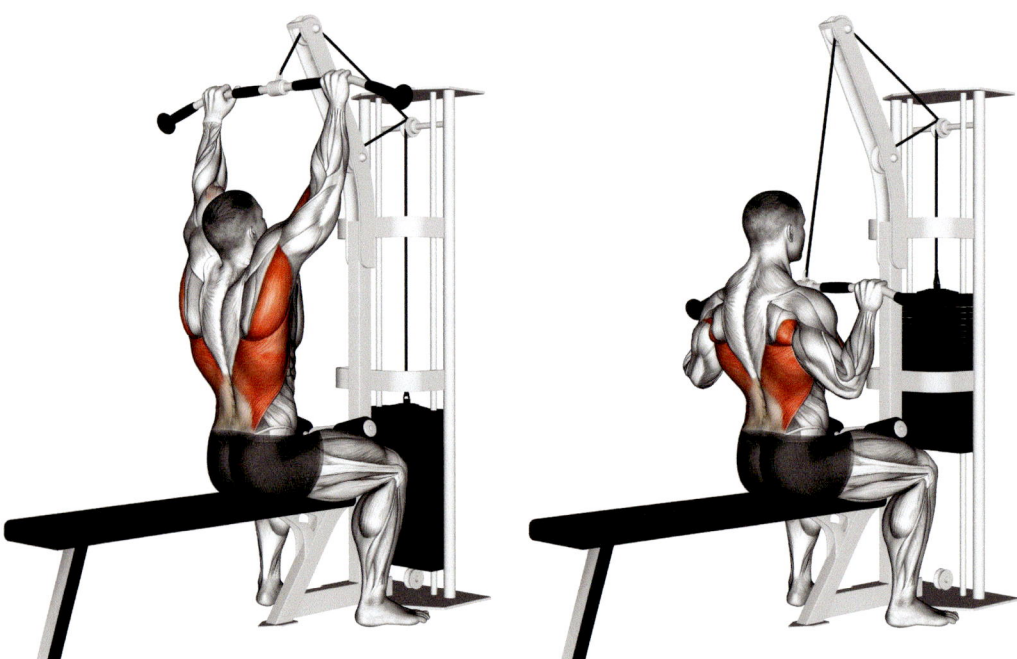

The illustration above shows the far superior lat pulldown technique, with the bar

DEVELOPMENT OF MY 100,000 SYSTEM

in front of the head, and the second illustration (below) shows the outdated, poor lat pulldown technique of pulling the bar behind the head and neck.

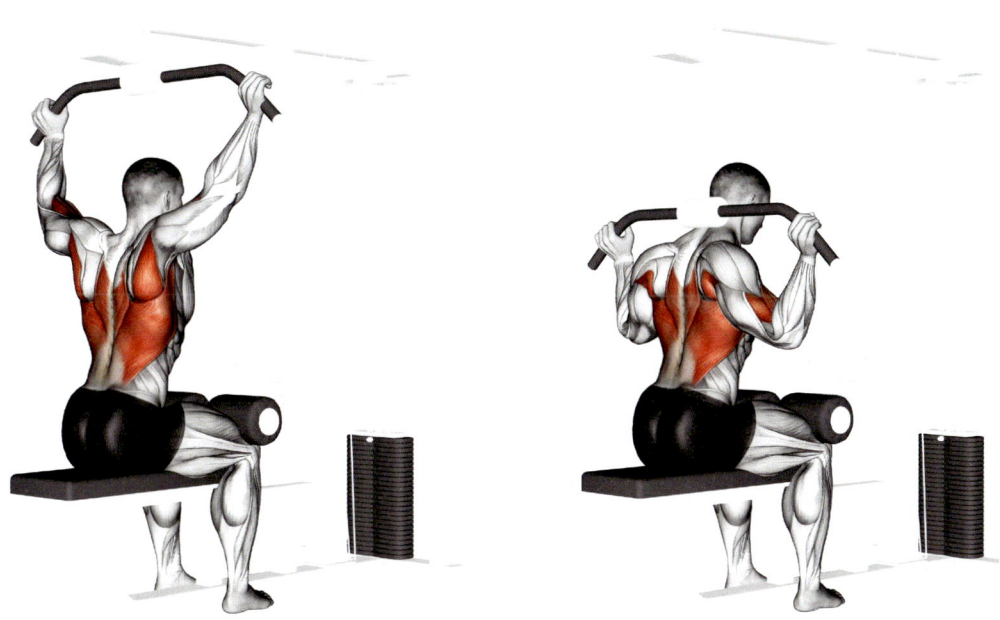

8. Back extensions (hyperextensions)

During my vast experience working with clients from all over the world, I have **never** seen this exercise performed correctly in any video, gym or exercise class.

The illustration below is a representation of the 'traditional' movement.

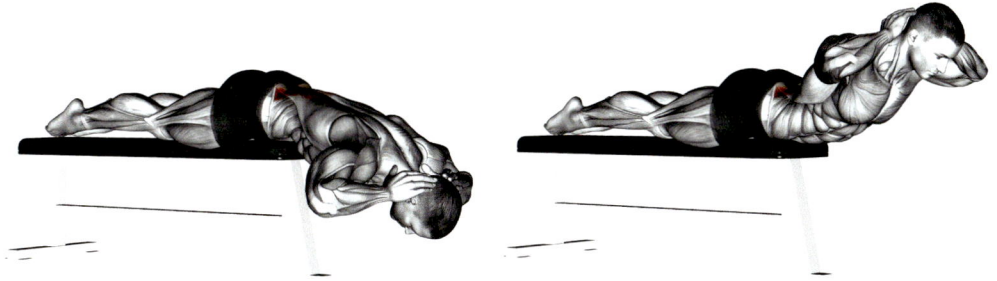

DEVELOPMENT OF MY 100,000 SYSTEM

Two main problems exist with the above technique. The vast majority of individuals lift the upper body far too high and too dynamically (fast). This results in significant back arching (hyperextension).

This issue, combined with the traditional hands behind the head position, just adds insult to injury (maybe literally). This loading or straining through the lower back muscles and joints, especially in a 'hyperextended' position, is simply unnecessary, and indeed, in my opinion, simply **wrong**.

A very easy modification changes this movement from being a highly controversial exercise into a great, highly effective strengthening, posture-enhancing exercise that more individuals should incorporate in their exercise routines.

The photograph below represents a lower back extension performed correctly.

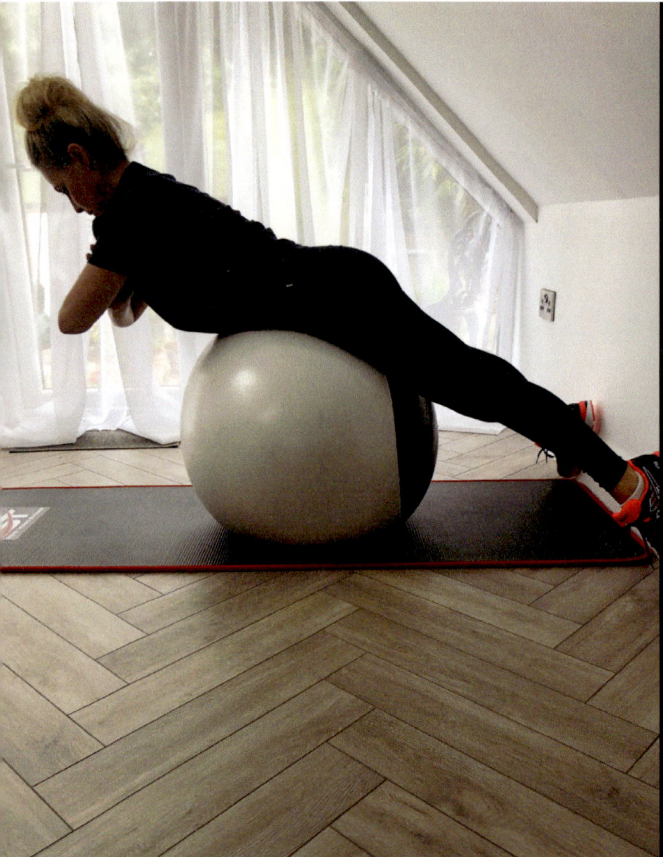

The use of a Swiss ball, with stability from the feet shoulder width apart and good body postural and spinal alignment, accompanied by the arms crossed in front of the chest, is the best way to perform lower back extensions, producing a highly efficient movement while maintaining musculoskeletal integrity.

My 100,000 system incorporates this modified version and other important lower spine conditioning exercises.

DEVELOPMENT OF MY 100,000 SYSTEM

9. Lunges

Standard lunges have been a mainstay of many exercise programmes for many years. Back in the late 1980s I introduced 'walking lunges' (ilustrated right) to my routines and to this day they are one of my favourite exercises. They do, however, need to be performed correctly.

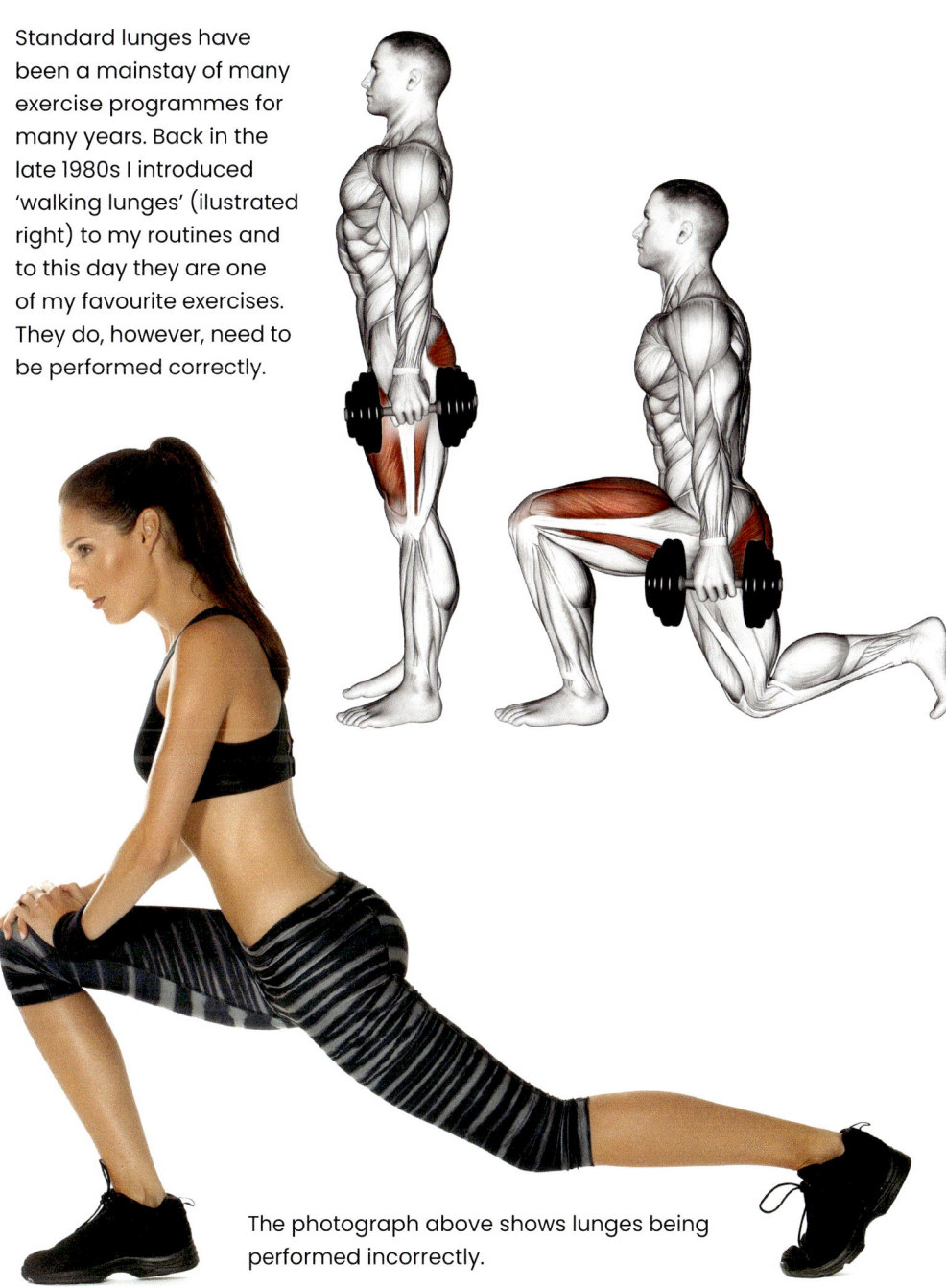

The photograph above shows lunges being performed incorrectly.

The FATHER FIGURE of FITNESS

DEVELOPMENT OF MY 100,000 SYSTEM

You will notice the forward lean of the torso (trunk), which encourages too much forward momentum of the whole body, with the front knee advancing beyond the line of the front foot and toes. This style is commonplace, and more importantly **wrong**.

Biomechanically speaking, some individuals find lunges technically challenging because of postural issues, spinal alignment and/or muscular tightness. Pursuing lunging with poor technique is neither sensible nor necessary. These individuals usually perform reverse, or backward, lunges (stepping backwards) with more comfort and hence, better technique – so this should be considered.

Whether you're performing traditional forward lunges or reverse lunges, good hip, knee and ankle/foot alignment is paramount. The photograph below shows how simple modifications can produce a technically perfect and good-quality lunge movement.

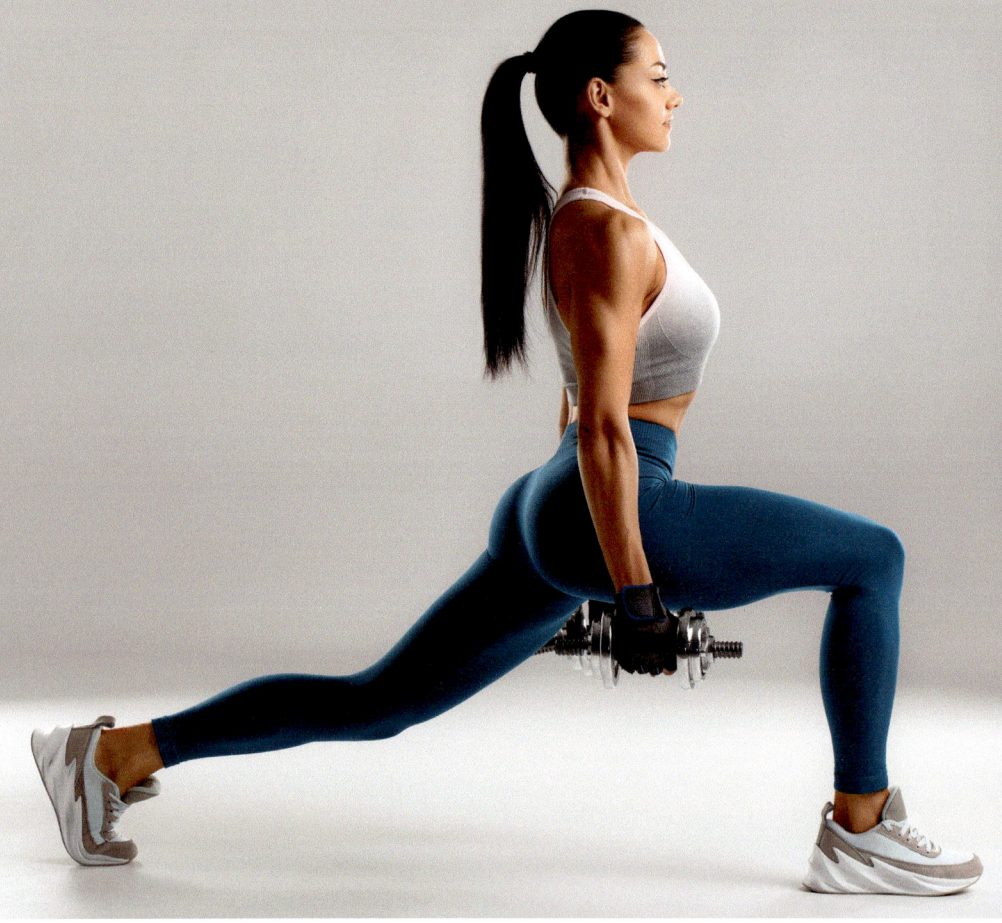

10. Deadlifts

This exercise has been another staple in exercise routines for many athletes, bodybuilders, sportsmen and sportswomen for decades. It is, however, a very controversial exercise, movement or position.

There are two opinions that are polar opposites. Many believe that this is a must-do exercise to achieve great all-around health, strength and fitness while, conversely, many believe that the deadlift is a seriously bad exercise for the human spine and should be avoided at all costs.

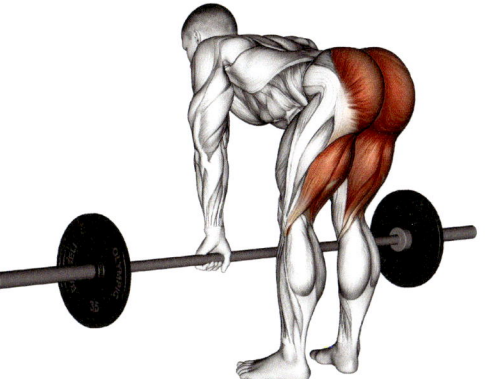

In fact, both of these opinions are incorrect. As a sport scientist, the true judgement of the effectiveness of this exercise lies in the science – the detail.

Above is an example of the traditional deadlift technique.

The key to this exercise again lies in its execution; its technique. You must either perform this movement correctly or not perform it at all. Bad technique, as shown (right), can put huge forces through the joints and discs in the lumbar spine (lower back), making the risk-reward ratio a very bad choice for most exercisers.

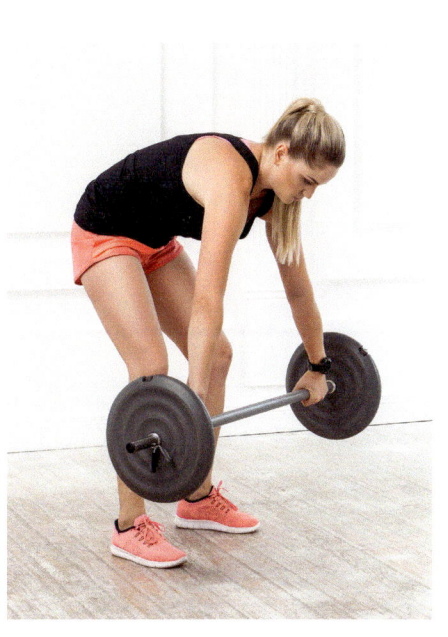

DEVELOPMENT OF MY 100,000 SYSTEM

If the deadlift is performed correctly, with well-rehearsed technique, it can be a major contributor to an individual's exercise regime. The correct technique involves the fine detail of:

a. Foot position – width, angle.
b. Hand position – width, grip.
c. Stabilising the thoracic spine – neutral/flat spine, engaging the core.
d. Engage the upper back (latissimus muscles), stabilising the shoulder girdles/thoracic spine.
e. Drive the hips and chest forward to lift the bar or weight.
f. Reverse the technique to lower the bar or weight.

This technique provides a great exercise for the whole body's posterior chain – the calves, hamstrings, glutes, lower, mid and upper back musculature, throughout the rear of the body.

However, this technique is not easy to establish, or specifically, maintain while using heavy weight. This technique is not just a matter of practice. – it simply **not** achievable for many individuals.

As I showed in previous chapters, we're all put together differently and we each have our own unique movement patterns. Many individuals have limb-length, joint range of movement and flexibility issues and biomechanical movement patterns that do not and will not lend themselves to this movement.

In summary, if you have good 'mechanics' and, hence, good technique, you can incorporate this exercise into your routines. However, unless you are an athlete, bodybuilder or super-fit sportsman or women, the risk-reward for this movement is simply not worth it. And that's why I do **not advocate** heavy deadlifts in my 100,000 programmes.

11. Barbell bent-over row

In the same vein as the deadlift exercise above, the barbell bent-over row is a highly contentious exercise, with two schools of thought lying on polar opposite sides of the exercising fence.

The illustration (top right) is an example of the traditional barbell bent-over row.

Once again, the correct technique involves the fine detail of foot, hand/grip position, the stabilisation of the thoracic (upper) and lumbar (lower) spine,

DEVELOPMENT OF MY 100,000 SYSTEM

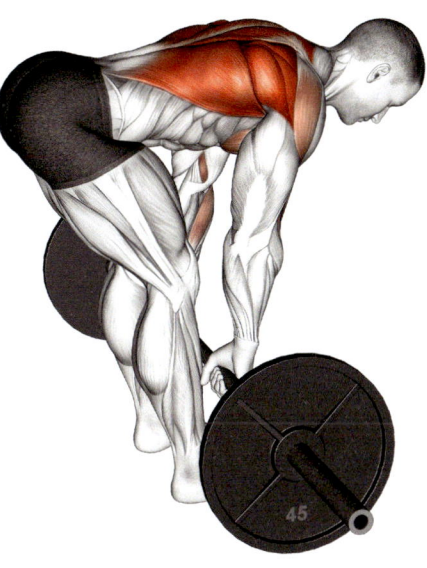 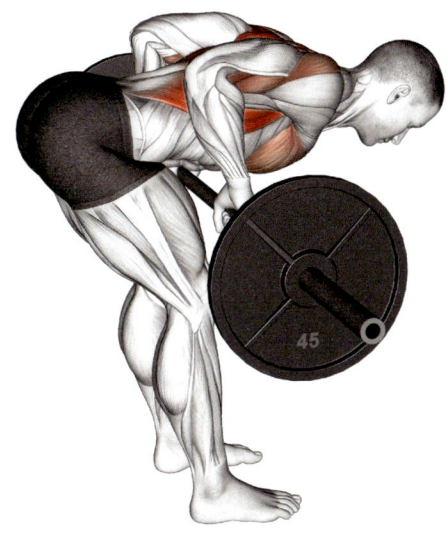

engaging the core correctly, adopting the correct knee angle, maintaining perfect balance and lifting the bar at the exact angle.

If an individual has the biomechanical ability to achieve this technique, and the consistency of repetition of this technique, then it may be proclaimed, as it is by many, as a master upper-back strengthening exercise.

The simple truth, however, is a repeat of my reasoning associated with the deadlift: correct technique is not just a matter of practice for many individuals. Limb length, joint range of movement and flexibility issues and biomechanical movement patterns do not and will not lend themselves to this movement. Sadly, poor technique is all too commonplace.

The photographs (left) depict the position, movement and technique that are all too familiar in gyms all around the world.

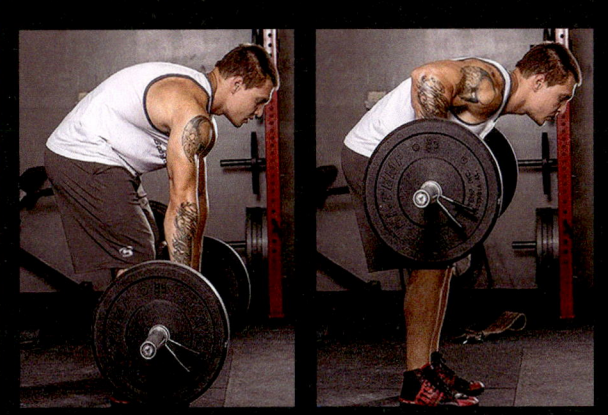

Poor technique doesn't just result in an ineffective exercise; it can overload the musculoskeletal system to the point of significant detriment to the spine and associated limbs and joints. So should you use this exercise?

Once again, in summary, if you have good mechanics and good technique, this exercise can be good for you. However, unless you are an athlete, bodybuilder or sportsman or woman, the risk-reward ratio for this exercise is simply not worth it. That is why I do not advocate this movement in my 100,000 system.

There are several other major issues that make the established way that we exercise **wrong**. Millions of individuals get into the habit of repeating their favourite exercises with their favourite body parts and routines – so much so that many exercisers constantly repeat the same exercise sessions time and time again. This one-dimensional approach to exercising produces, at best, a one-dimensional result.

As a sport scientist, I am acutely aware that the human body functions at its best with a variety of multi-directional, coordinated, fluid, multi-segmental movement patterns, and it therefore needs to be exercised as closely as possible to this organic need for variety of movement.

So exercise routines must be different each time you train, and they must be packed with a significant variety and blend of movements and exercises.

During my 37-year career I have **never** given the same client, even those with whom I've worked closely continuously over many years, the same routine twice. Every session is different from the last one and different from the next one. This variety keeps the body guessing and on its toes, and keeps the exerciser mentally alert and engaged.

The main reason for this obsession with variety is that it **works** – it keeps the body progressing with each and every new, different position, movement or exercise. That's why my 100,000 system – 900 exercises that can be juggled around to ensure that you never do the same exercise routine twice – has variety at its heart.

You must **stop** just doing your favourite exercises – **stop** just concentrating on the exercises you are good at and **stop** just exercising your best muscle groups. You must *start* doing the exercises that you don't like, are not good at or have never done before.

DEVELOPMENT OF MY 100,000 SYSTEM

YOUR BODY NEEDS CONTINUED VARIETY OF EXERCISE. This is my **Golden Rule Number Six**.

The next major issue that must change is our obsessive belief that we must work towards a defined number of repetitions on each and every exercise set. Please remember that our muscles cannot count, and we must learn to **stop** counting.

I understand and appreciate that a target number of repetitions in a set has some general credibility, especially for beginners, but any experienced exerciser will know that no two repetitions or sets of exercises are ever perfectly the same, so just reaching your ten, 15 or 20 reps target and then ceasing must simply **stop** being the accepted norm.

Adhering to this 'norm' misses out on the most important repetitions of all – those that produce the muscular fatigue that makes all the difference to our progress. After all, the main purpose of repetitions is the achievement of the desired level of intensity and fatigue. The current belief is still that gentle fatigue (light weights or resistance) over a higher number of reps (20 to 30) equates to a muscle endurance effect; moderate fatigue (medium weights or resistance) over a medium number of reps (15 to 20), equates to a muscle-toning effect; and high levels of fatigue (heavy weights or resistance) over a low number of reps equates to increased muscle strength and size.

This belief has been the norm for decades, but the reality is it's **wrong**, nothing short of rubbish, outdated and scientifically incorrect.

For muscles to respond as quickly as possible, they need variety – they need low reps, medium reps and high reps. Muscles also need variety of resistance/weight – low, medium and high. Importantly, irrespective of weight/resistance, sets of isolation exercises should **never** be dictated by numbers but by levels of fatigue. And the only way to judge fatigue is to f***eel/experience fatigue, feel/experience the movement***.

Judging all exercises by **feel** or **experience** is a major missing link in the world of exercise. This feeling and experiencing the movement is called PROPRIOCEPTION.

Technique is very important and the starting point to all exercises, but it's also crucial not just to focus on what you are doing, but also on **what you are feeling**. The best way to do this is to close your eyes, listen and learn – learn to focus on the 'feeling' of the movement. This will allow you to tune in to your muscle, your position and your movement, allowing you to 'feel' the muscle lengthening, 'feel' the muscle shortening/contracting and 'feel' the muscle fatiguing.

By feeling your exercises this way, you will automatically focus away from simply counting your reps or allowing your mind to wander. This proprioceptive tuning-in – feeling, experiencing a muscle and/or movement – is simply the best way to exercise. If you can learn to feel and experience each and every exercise, you will progress faster than ever.

I have always put an enormous amount of emphasis on understanding, learning and rehearsing all exercises with the eyes closed, to allow the body to develop its proprioceptive abilities – to enhance the mind-muscle connection and focus away from counting numbers.

My next **Golden Rule, Number Seven** is, therefore:

1. Choose your weight/resistance.
2. **Close your eyes**.
3. Ensure slow and controlled technique.
4. **Focus, find, feel, fatigue** your muscles and movements.

Finding, feeling, experiencing your exercises in your mind's eye is crucial. It is another fundamental missing link in how the world exercises, and it is really the only way to know that you are carrying out your movements and exercises correctly and productively.

Once you have 'found' your muscle, this is the starting point of your set. When you are highly focussed, your eyes are closed and your technique is great, you may 'find' your muscle after just two or three reps. However, you will do many, many sets in which you just can't 'find' your muscle until rep ten, or 12, 14 or even 20.

Once you have 'found' your muscle you must stay focused, keep the 'feeling', keep the repetitions smooth and fatigue will set in as it never has before. When fatigue starts to set in, the muscle produces lactic acid, which builds up in the muscle, and you will experience a burning sensation. This sensation is imperative in the toning and strengthening of your muscles. Stopping a set of repetitions before experiencing this burning sensation just because you have reached your desired number of reps is simply **wrong**.

This analogy explains why counting numbers doesn't always work. Sets of repetitions need to be judged by feeling, by burning, by fatigue and **not** by numbers.

DEVELOPMENT OF MY 100,000 SYSTEM

To respond to exercises, muscles need to be taken out of their comfort zone. The feeling, hence fatigue, hence burning sensation of an exercise is exactly what is needed to do this. In essence, no feeling, no fatigue, no burning equals no progression. Muscle fatigue (burning) doesn't just come from heavy weights, hard work and effort, it comes from quality. Finding, feeling, experiencing each movement is the **best** way to achieve quality of movement, quality of exercise.

To summarise – **Golden Rule Number Seven** is CLOSE YOUR EYES and FOCUS, FIND, FEEL and FATIGUE.

Having addressed all of the major issues that individuals continually get wrong, and having modified certain positions, exercises and movements to make them safer and kinder to your muscles, bones and joints, my next challenge in developing my 100,000 system was to incorporate the plethora of exercises, positions, stretches, stability movements, joint and body part issues that have been completely missed or forgotten about in almost all other exercise regimes.

I have used, tried and tested these missing ingredients with hundreds of individuals over many decades, and it has shown me – and more importantly, proved to them – that these positions, movements and exercises are vital to achieve the variety, versatility and the balance of exercises needed for comprehensive exercise routines that produce balanced results. The experience of working with hundreds of clients from all over the world has shown me that hardly anyone understands, or has been taught, the importance of hip/pelvic function and the importance of its associated musculature – the gluteals.

Very few individuals have been taught or shown the importance of the shoulder girdle/joint position and function, or even heard of the importance of the shoulder rotator cuff musculature.

Similarly, the importance of foot, ankle and lower leg position, function and musculature is nowhere to be seen and I have **never** come across anyone who has ever heard of nerve stretching, flossing or gliding, let alone anyone who knows how to perform these important stretches correctly.

In more than 100,000 one-to-one personal training sessions I have only come across a few isolated instances where an individual has used different muscle contraction exercises or techniques (concentric, isometric and/or eccentric muscle contractions), and/or muscle activation exercises.

Also of great importance here is the subject of the back/spine and the core/

DEVELOPMENT OF MY 100,000 SYSTEM

abdominal area. Individuals are more interested in these two areas than any other. These two topics are the most discussed and most disputed, with more speculation, myths and misinformed opinion than any other. I receive more questions about them than any other subject, and yet very few individuals seem to understand what they should and should not do.

Let's consider some of these missing links in more detail.

1. Hips/pelvis/gluteal muscles

Let me start by stating the obvious. As human beings we move on two legs and these legs join the body or trunk at the hips or pelvis. The hips/pelvis therefore, 'geographically' speaking, are enormously important, providing as they do great stability and mechanical and functional strength to the entire body, both below (the legs) and above (spine, ribs, head, neck and shoulders).

The major muscle group that surrounds this area is composed of the gluteals (gluteus maximus, gluteus medius and gluteus minimus). This muscle group is relatively large for a very good reason: it is **very, very important**.

Below is an illustration of gluteal anatomy.

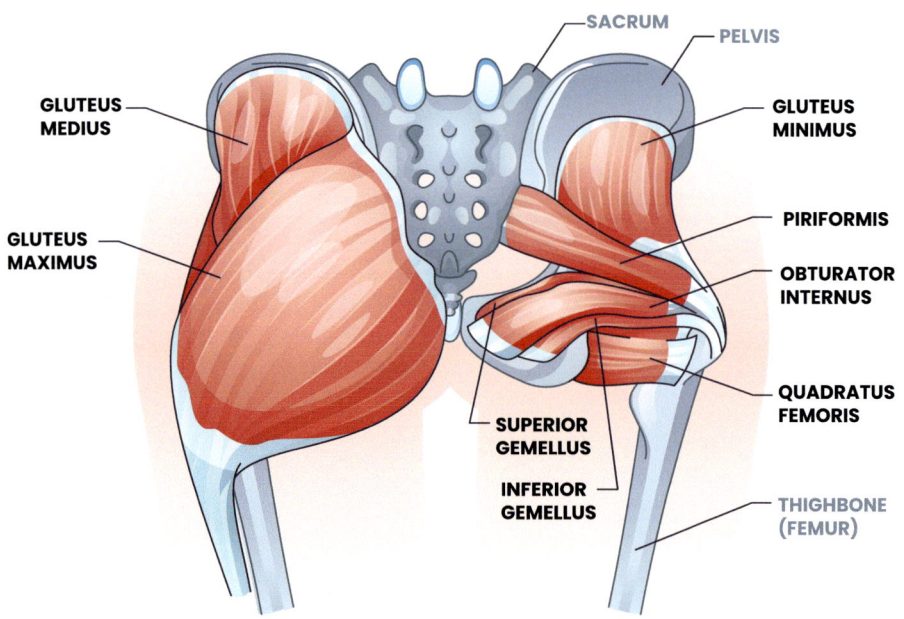

DEVELOPMENT OF MY 100,000 SYSTEM

The hips, pelvis and gluteals provide the foundational support and strength for the human spine. The gluteals are therefore critical to human biomechanics.

It is true that a number of traditional gym exercises (such as squats and lunges) should utilise these important gluteal muscles, but the harsh reality is that many individuals have gluteal muscles that are tight and weak and barely function at all, and certainly not to the degree necessary to control, aid or enhance their biomechanics, support the vulnerable spine and manage their aches and pains. I have therefore flooded my 100,000 system with the best specific and all-round gluteal exercises.

Here, I want to address specifically what in my opinion is a missing link and a priority for you to incorporate immediately into your routines. The gluteus medius is vital to human movement and function, yet hardly anyone seems to have heard of it, let alone know where it is, what it does or how to test, stretch or exercise it properly. It is a major forgotten muscle. Below is a photograph of the gluteus medius anatomy.

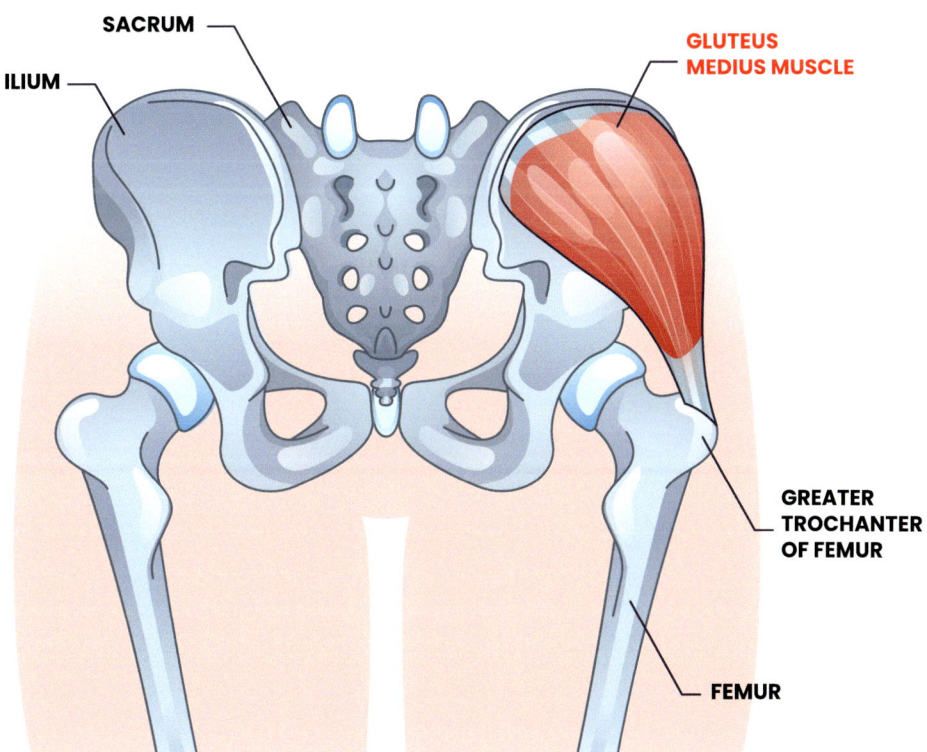

DEVELOPMENT OF MY 100,000 SYSTEM

Functions of the gluteus medius:

- Abduction of the hip (lifting the leg up to the side).
- Flexion of the hip (lifting the knee up towards the chest).
- Internal and external rotation of the thigh.
- Provides stability to the pelvis.

To test for a weak gluteus medius, attempt a one-leg squat. If the opposite hip drops, the gluteus medius is weak, as seen in the photograph below.

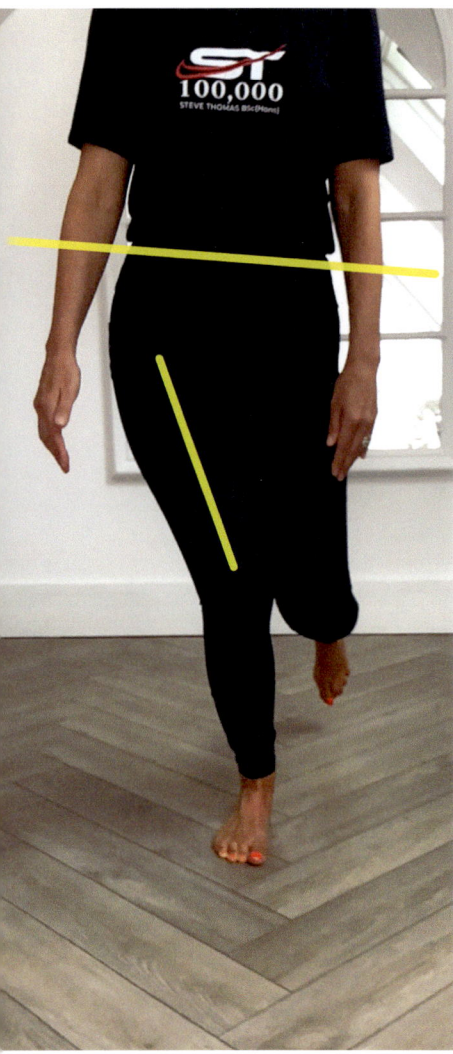

As I have stated, poor knee and hip functioning results from both weakness and tightness of the gluteus medius. It is therefore imperative to stretch it regularly. I have included a whole range of the best GM stretches into my programmes, and the example below is my favourite – and one that hardly anyone else seems to employ.

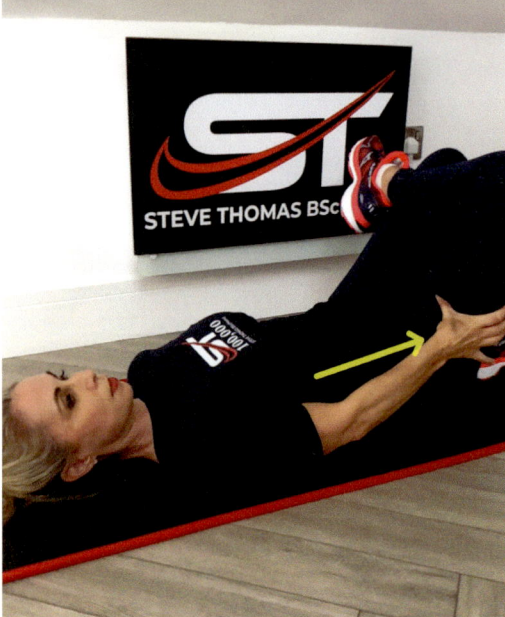

This is not the standard 'cross-over' gluteal stretch. Perform this as follows:

a. Cross one leg over the other – placing the mid lower leg (not the foot) on the opposite knee.
b. Push the upper leg (not the knee) away from the hip, as shown by the arrow.

This stretch really lengthens the GM and I have found it to be extremely productive.

Exercising/strengthening the gluteus medius

My 100,000 system is jam-packed with the best gluteus medius exercises and an example is below.

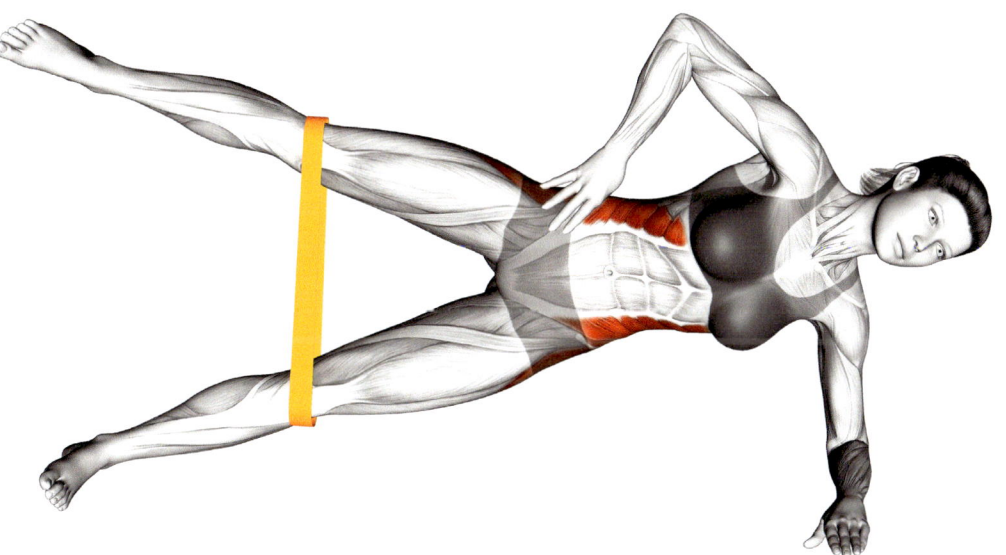

The strength and functioning capabilities of the gluteus medius are inhibited by many everyday positions, activities and movements, such as sleeping continuously on one side, standing repeatedly with all our bodyweight through one leg and continually crossing our legs. Weakness of this vital muscle leads to potential injury of the hip, thigh, knee and ankle.

Therefore in summary, **every** single one of us **must** exercise this vastly important muscle.

DEVELOPMENT OF MY 100,000 SYSTEM

2. Shoulder stability – the rotator cuff muscles

The shoulder girdle/joint is a multifaceted, multifunctional and multidirectional joint like no other. As a ball and socket joint it is quite magnificent in its range of movement. It is the most mobile joint in the human body and this mobility allows for:

a. Abduction – moving the arm away to the side of the body
b. Adduction – moving the arm inwards and across the midline of the body
c. Flexion – raising the arm forward and upwards
d. Extension – moving the arm downwards and backwards
e. Internal rotation – rotating the hand (thumb) inwards
f. External rotation – rotating the hand (thumb) outwards
g. 360 degrees circumduction – full 360-degree rotation
h. Protraction – pulling the shoulder girdle forwards
i. Retraction – pulling the shoulder girdle backwards
j. Elevation – lifting the shoulder girdle
k. Depression – lowering the shoulder girdle.

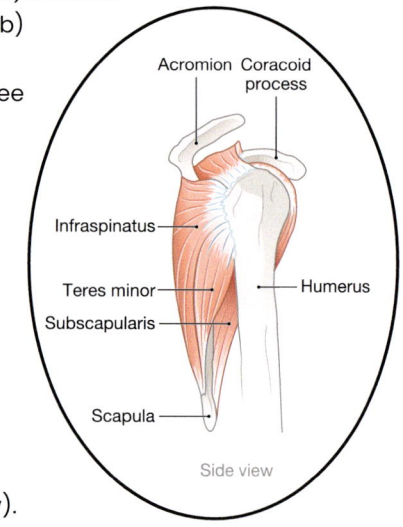

The trade-off for such a variety of movement is, however, **instability**. This inherent instability is compensated for by the rotator cuff muscles, ligaments and tendons, shown (right and below).

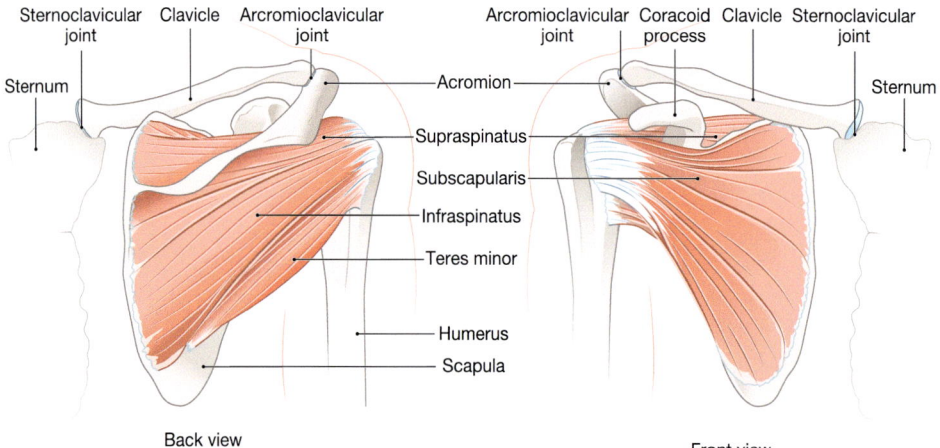

DEVELOPMENT OF MY 100,000 SYSTEM

The modern-day practice of sitting for hours in front of a computer screen or staring at a mobile phone can cause rotator cuff issues. The enormous stresses and strains that we inflict on the shoulder joint/girdle with activities like swimming, throwing, lifting, boxing, judo, volleyball, rugby, rowing, baseball, cricket, golf, tennis, squash, badminton, table tennis, basketball and so on add to the sheer volume and load that the shoulder endures during so many traditional gym exercises like press-ups, bench presses, chest flies, shoulder presses, lateral raises, dips and deadlifts.

It becomes abundantly clear that for functional support and stability, a proper understanding of how to test, stretch and strengthen the rotator cuff musculature is absolutely essential for each and every one of us.

A simple test to see if you have rotator cuff/shoulder girdle stiffness, lack of flexibility or range of movement is the Aspley scratch test, as follows.

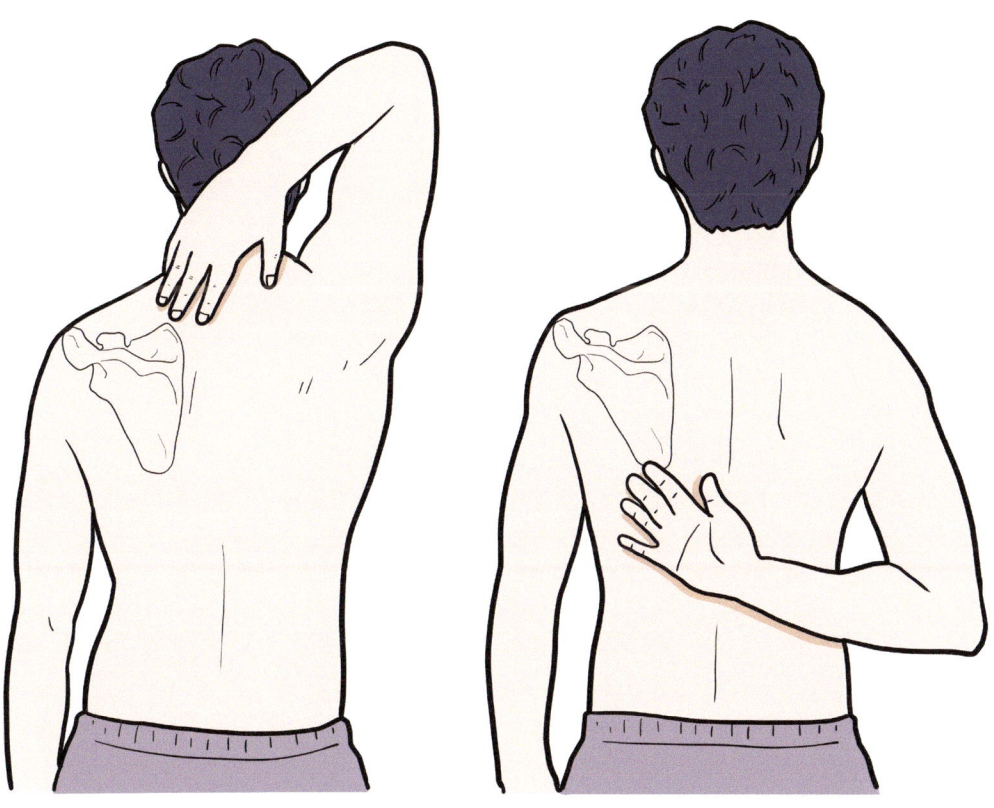

DEVELOPMENT OF MY 100,000 SYSTEM

Often called swimmer's shoulder, untreated rotator cuff issues lead to shoulder impingement syndrome, which is **all** too common for regular exercisers, gym-goers, sportsmen and women. Shoulder impingement syndrome (SIS) is depicted below.

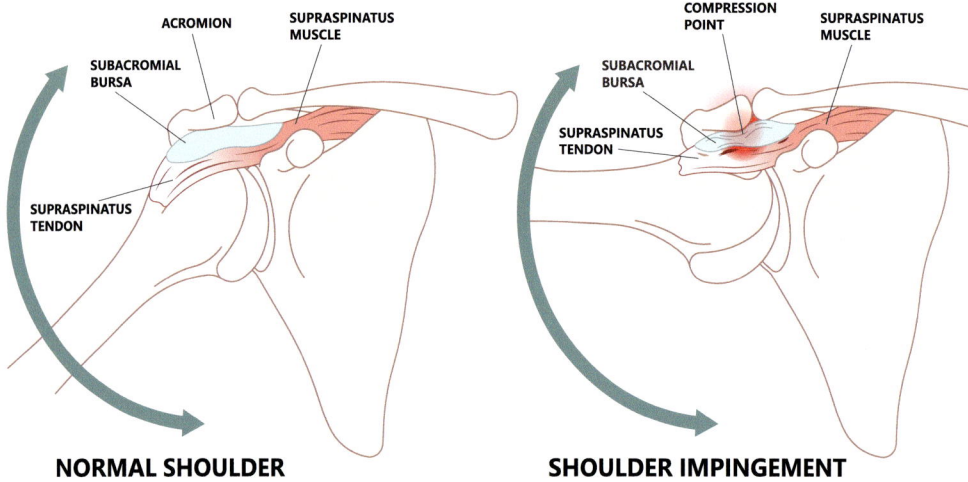

NORMAL SHOULDER **SHOULDER IMPINGEMENT**

SIS is looming for all of us if we don't respect the importance of rotator cuff exercises. I strongly advise all individuals to perform rotator cuff exercises, so my 100,000 system includes the best ones, an example of which is below.

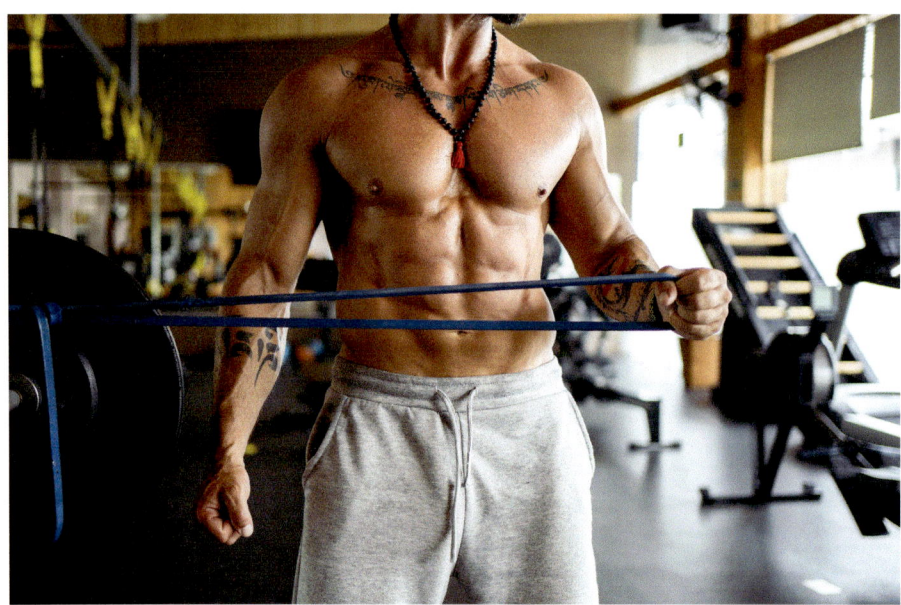

3. Foot/ankle/lower leg stability

When was the last time you exercised your feet? When was the last time you exercised your ankles? Have you ever stretched or exercised your soleus (lower rear leg) muscle? What about your tibialis anterior (shin) muscle? As I thought: probably not.

As I mentioned earlier, considering that we are human beings that locomote on two legs, very little attention is ever given to exercising or stretching our feet, ankles and lower leg musculature. Below is an illustration of our lower leg anatomy.

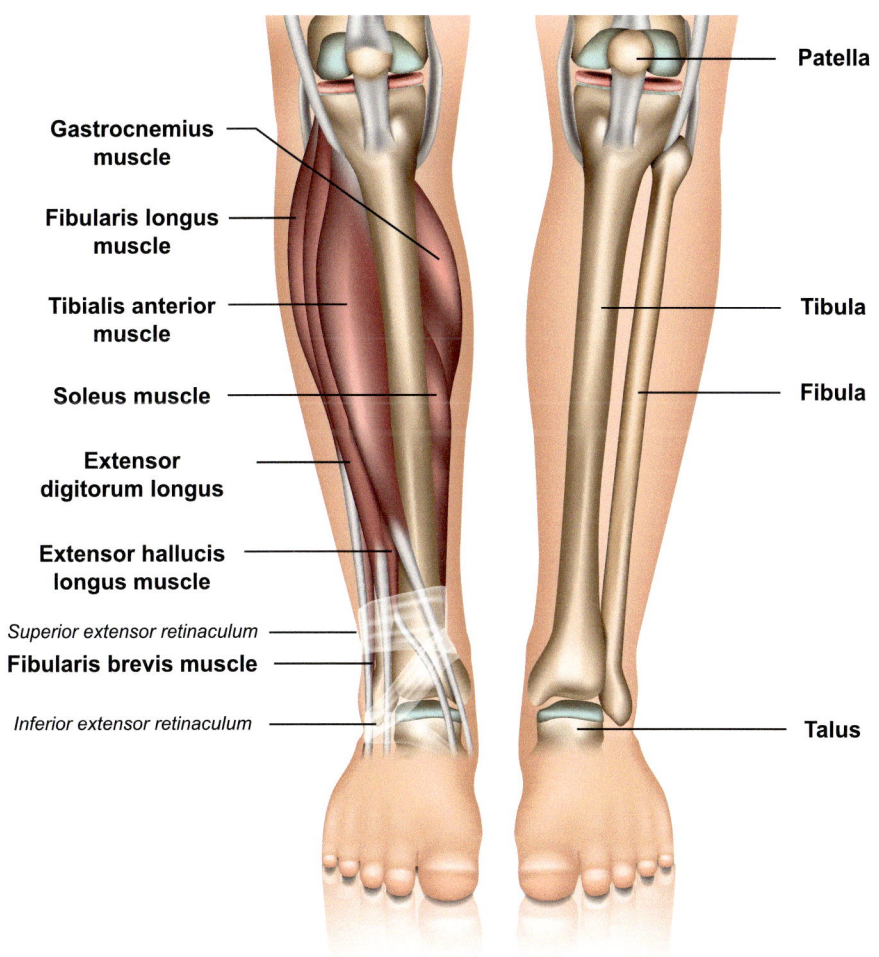

DEVELOPMENT OF MY 100,000 SYSTEM

As they're the first line of defence against significant ground reaction forces that reverberate up the body during walking, jogging, running and all major activities, the position, flexibility, strength and stability of our feet, ankles and lower legs are paramount in the human body's biomechanics, and yet very little attention is given to these vital components in exercise programmes.

The missing elements of lower leg training are as follows.

   a. Balance/proprioception/stability training.

Everyone should carry out the simple SLB (standing leg balance) test. Simply stand on one leg without shoes on and close your eyes for ten seconds to see if you can maintain your balance. You will be amazed as to how difficult this is – often much more difficult on one leg than the other. I have tested thousands of individuals with this simple test and it is quite extraordinary how many individuals can't do this for three or four seconds, let alone ten.

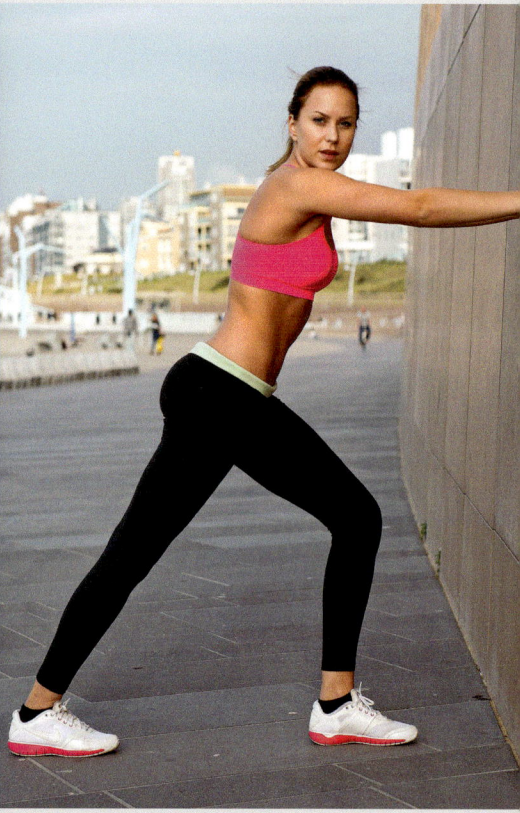

Balance training to aid both proprioception and joint stability is therefore essential for good human biomechanics and should be incorporated into all of our training routines. I include a whole variety of these exercises in all my programmes.

   b. Correct stretching of the musculature.

As with any skeletal muscle, correct stretching is paramount in our training, and the less 'glamorous' lower leg muscles are no exception. The calf muscle group consists of the gastrocnemius and soleus muscles. The standard calf stretch (see right), is predominantly for the gastrocnemius muscle.

DEVELOPMENT OF MY 100,000 SYSTEM

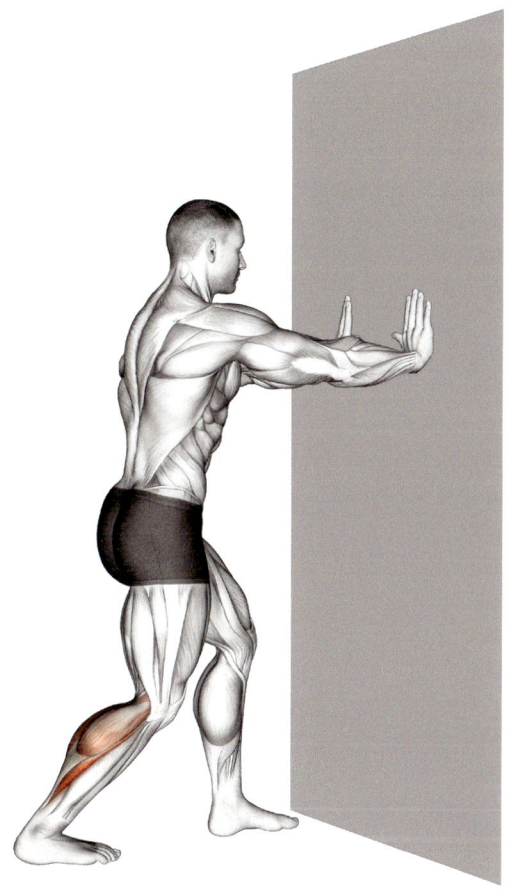

Specifically, the soleus remains a muscle that is rarely stretched correctly if it is stretched at all. The instruction for how to stretch the soleus (see left) seems quite straightforward, but many individuals struggle to 'feel' the stretch significantly, sufficiently or indeed correctly.

Stretching the soleus muscle is essential not only directly but also indirectly in aiding foot mechanics and hence the biomechanical chain. Everyone must practise this position until they can really 'feel' the stretch correctly and consistently. Variations of this stretch are included in my 100,000 system.

c. Correct exercising of the musculature

Correct exercising of the lower leg musculature must consist of much greater variety of exercises than just performing the traditional calf raise. Exercising the soleus, peroneus and tibialis muscles are of equal importance, and an example can be seen below.

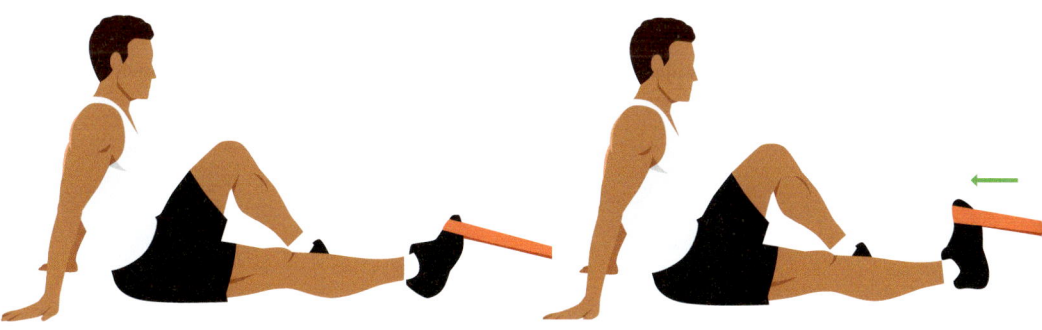

DEVELOPMENT OF MY 100,000 SYSTEM

A complete variety of lower leg exercises is included in my 100,000 system.

    d. Ankle mobility exercises

A simple test for the range of movement (mobility) of the ankle joint is the weight-bearing lunge test (WBLT) or the dorsiflexion lunge test (DFT), as depicted right.

Place one foot as far away from the wall as possible, ensuring that the knee can just touch the wall. Measure the distance from the wall. Every centimetre correlates with 3.6 degrees of ankle dorsiflexion (mobility). Ideally the toes should be 2-4 inches away from the wall.

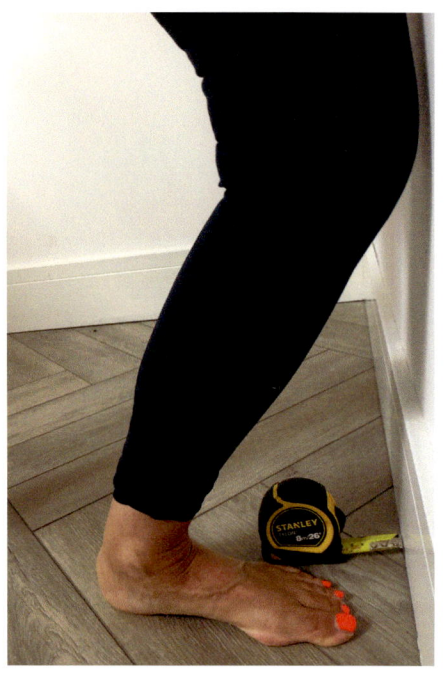

My experience has shown me that lack of ankle mobility is a much more frequent occurrence than one would ever believe, and mobility movements therefore feature heavily in my 100,000 system. Even a simple ankle circle exercise, as shown below, can maintain, boost or enhance ankle mobility.

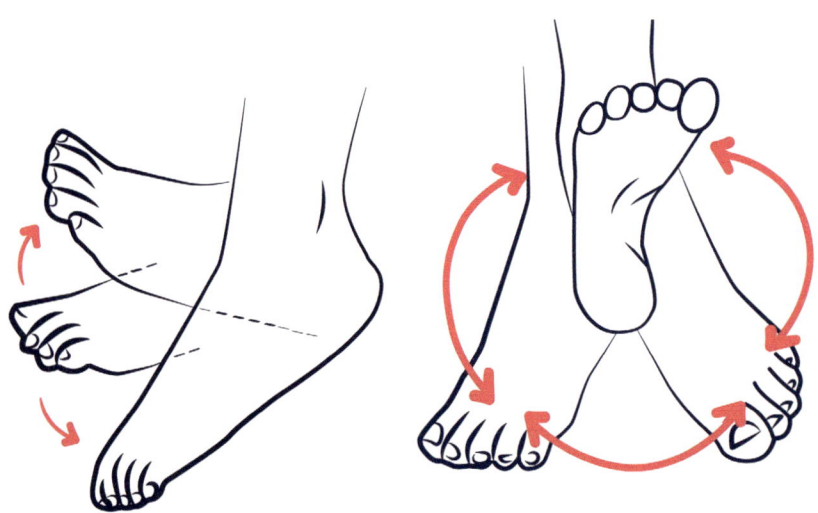

DEVELOPMENT OF MY 100,000 SYSTEM

4. Nerve stretching/gliding/flossing

The human nervous system is a highly complex component of the human body. It consists of the central nervous system (CNS) and the peripheral nervous system (PNS) and essentially acts as our in-built computer, the brain being the software and the nerves being the hardware.

It has four main functions:

1. Voluntary control of movement.
2. Control of the body's internal environment to maintain homeostasis.
3. Programming of spinal cord reflexes.
4. Memory and learning.

From an exercising perspective, if the PNS is compromised then all exercises, movements, activities and sports are compromised.

Nerve testing and nerve 'stretching' has traditionally only been the domain for physiotherapy, osteopathy and chiropractic treatment and seem never to have been used in the general or specific exercising or sporting worlds. My experience has shown me that incorporating some very easy and gentle nerve 'stretching' or mobilisation techniques, increasing range of motion and reducing pain, can be very beneficial to many individuals.

A simple example is shown below.

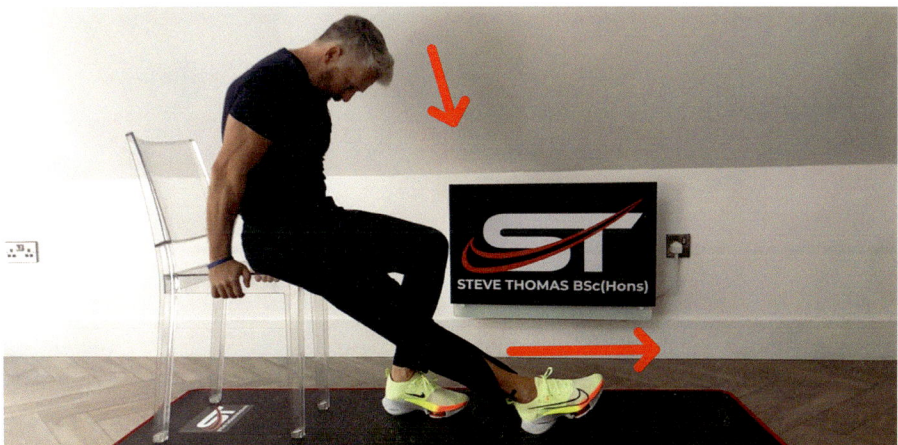

I advocate the use of both upper and lower limb nerve mobilisation exercises and include many variations in my 100,000 system.

The FATHER FIGURE of FITNESS

DEVELOPMENT OF MY 100,000 SYSTEM

5. Different muscle contraction exercises

I need to divide this element into two main sections, as follows.

   a. Activation muscle contraction exercises.

Activation exercises are short isolation exercises that essentially 'jump-start' muscles. These simple exercises prepare muscles for the more intense cardiovascular, weight training, gym and sporting exercises by increasing blood flow to the isolated muscle.

These exercises should form a valuable part of a complete warm-up routine. They are also vital in training or rehearsing the **mind-body** connection – a skill that many individuals simply do **not** possess.

They are slow, mild, easy and gentle exercises that focus on the 'feeling' of the movements and muscles and can dramatically increase your quality and efficiency of movement, encouraging and enhancing your ability to get stronger and progress quicker.

Many exercisers may see these exercises as a time-wasting distraction from the real hard work of 'proper' exercising. On the contrary, remembering that quality outstrips everything, the increase in quality of your exercising as a result of doing these activation exercises will propel your results like never before. In my 100,000 system I have incorporated many activation exercises for the

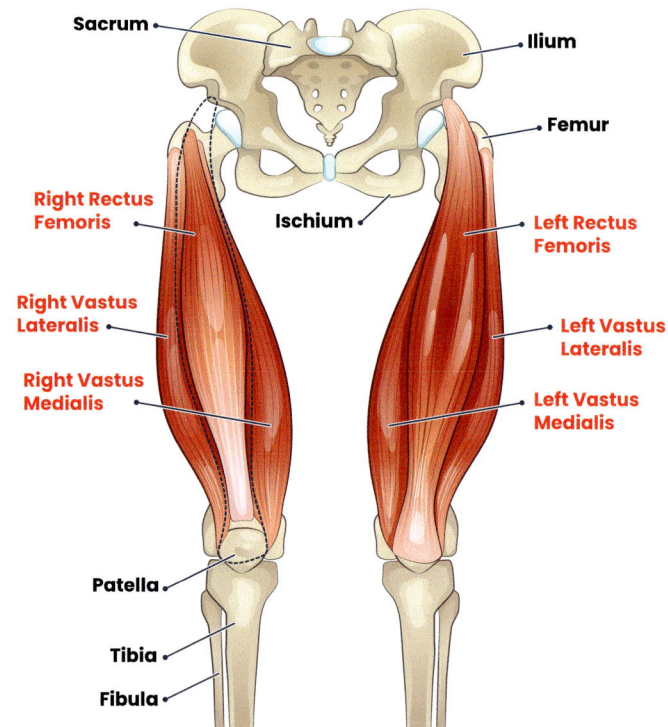

DEVELOPMENT OF MY 100,000 SYSTEM

entire musculoskeletal system.

Below is an example, and one of my favourite exercises that doubles up as a knee rehabilitation exercise. There are no miracle exercises, but this comes as close as is possible as it relieves a multitude of knee complaints, aches, pains and injuries.

This exercise is for the vastus medialis (see diagram bottom left), which forms one part of the quadricep (front thigh) muscle and is often called the tear drop muscle or the VMO (vastus medialis oblique).

The activation exercise for this muscle is as follows.

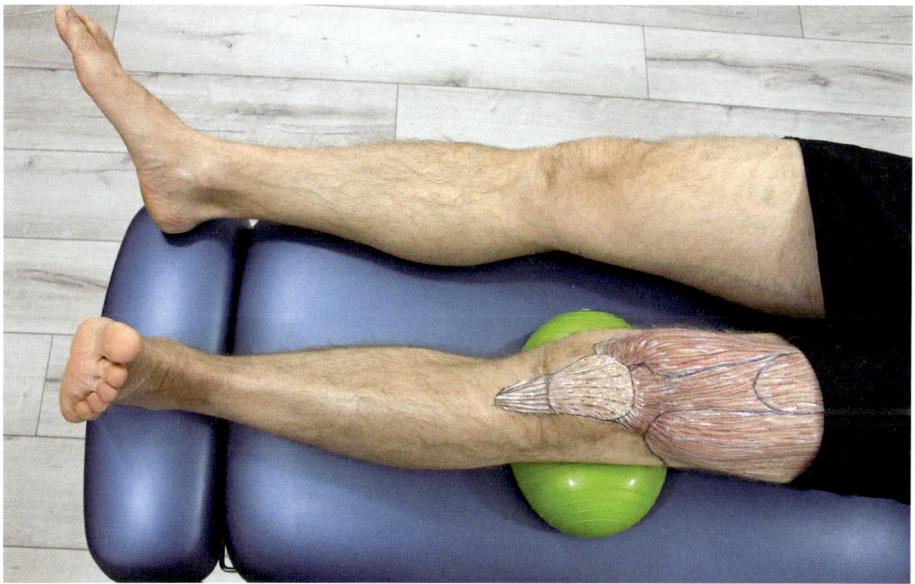

For this exercise I advocate **activating, flexing and squeezing** the VMO, pushing the knee joint downwards, holding for one second, then releasing and repeating for 50 or even 100 repetitions.

Activation exercises for the entire body are very much a missing component in almost all exercise, gym and sporting routines and hence why I include them in each and every one of my routines.

   b. Concentric/eccentric/isometric contraction exercises.

DEVELOPMENT OF MY 100,000 SYSTEM

There are three types of skeletal muscle contractions: a) concentric, b) eccentric and c) isometric, as depicted below.

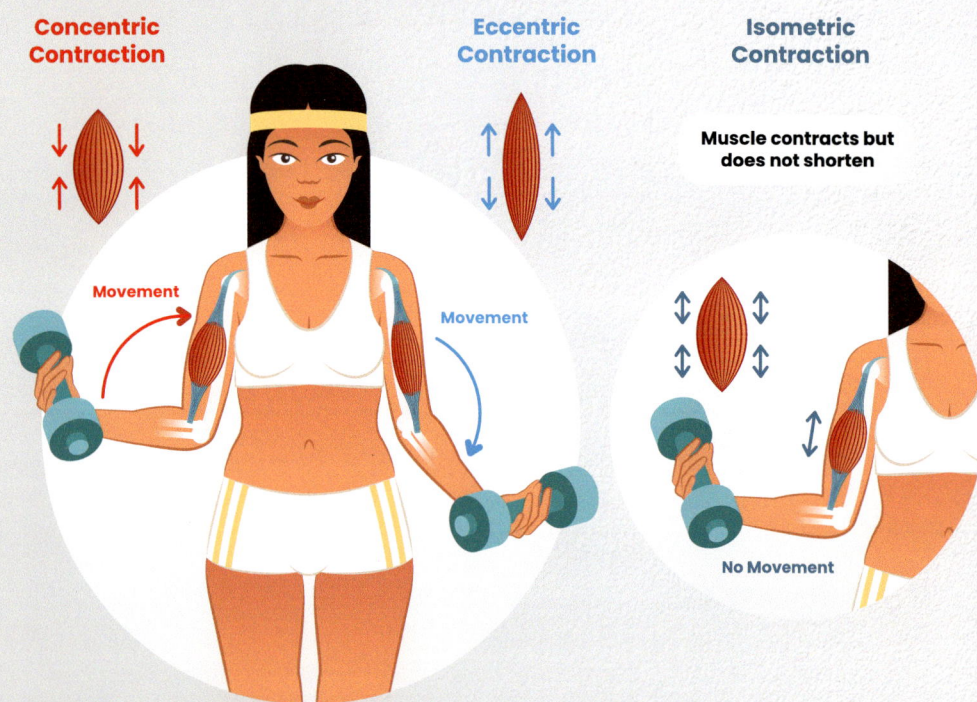

Traditional exercising predominantly uses concentric contractions to attempt to fatigue the muscles to the desired degree.

It's a mystery to me why so few teachers, coaches and trainers fail to adopt eccentric **or** isometric exercises into their routines. These other contractions are not solely for elite athletes, sportsmen and women; **you** should incorporate isometric and eccentric muscle contraction exercises into your training routines. Simple and easy to do, they will also provide the increased variety of exercise that is so badly lacking in most individuals' training routines.

The 'wall sit' exercise, (shown right), is a great example of an isometric exercise.

DEVELOPMENT OF MY 100,000 SYSTEM

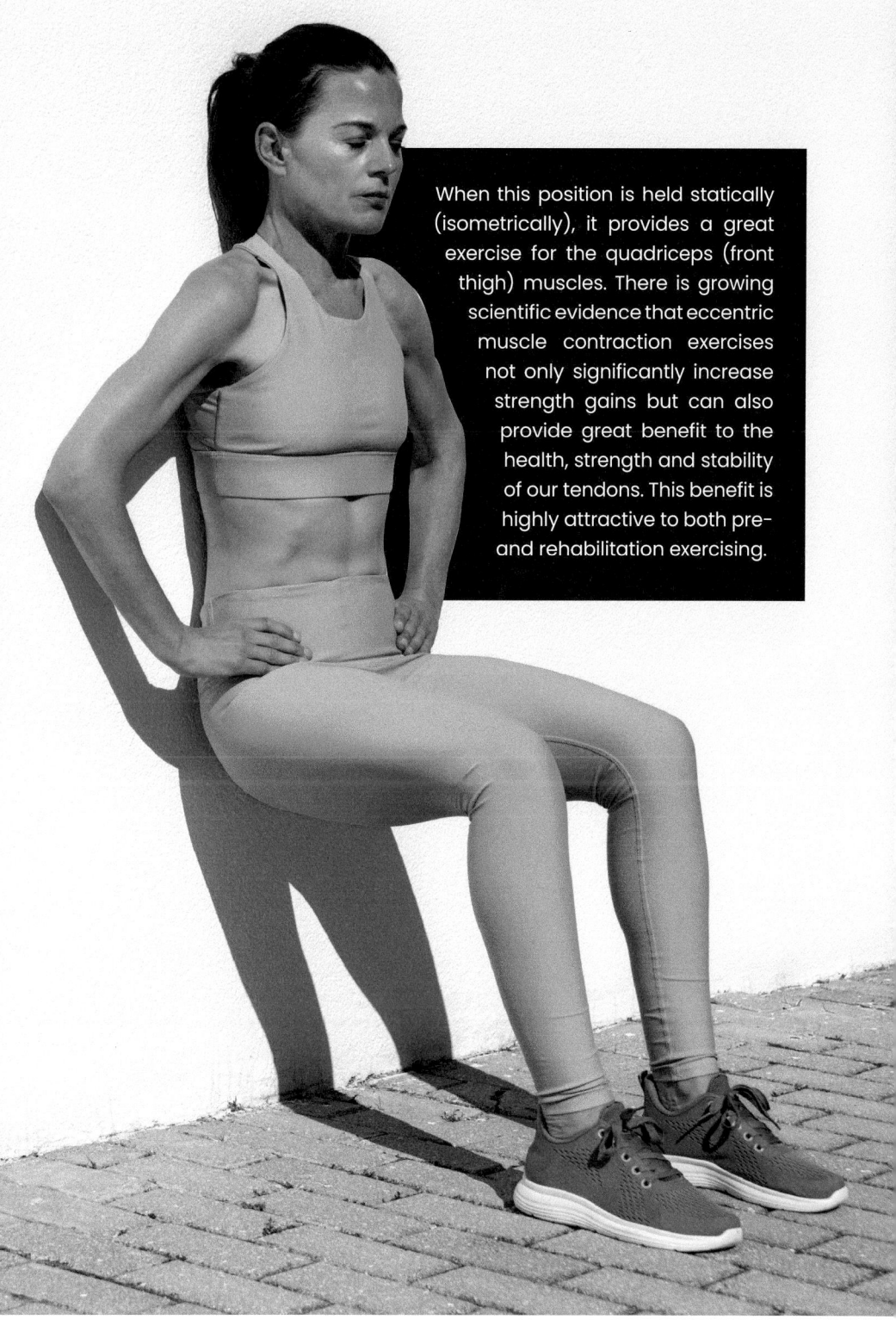

When this position is held statically (isometrically), it provides a great exercise for the quadriceps (front thigh) muscles. There is growing scientific evidence that eccentric muscle contraction exercises not only significantly increase strength gains but can also provide great benefit to the health, strength and stability of our tendons. This benefit is highly attractive to both pre- and rehabilitation exercising.

DEVELOPMENT OF MY 100,000 SYSTEM

The photograph below is a good example of an eccentric exercise.

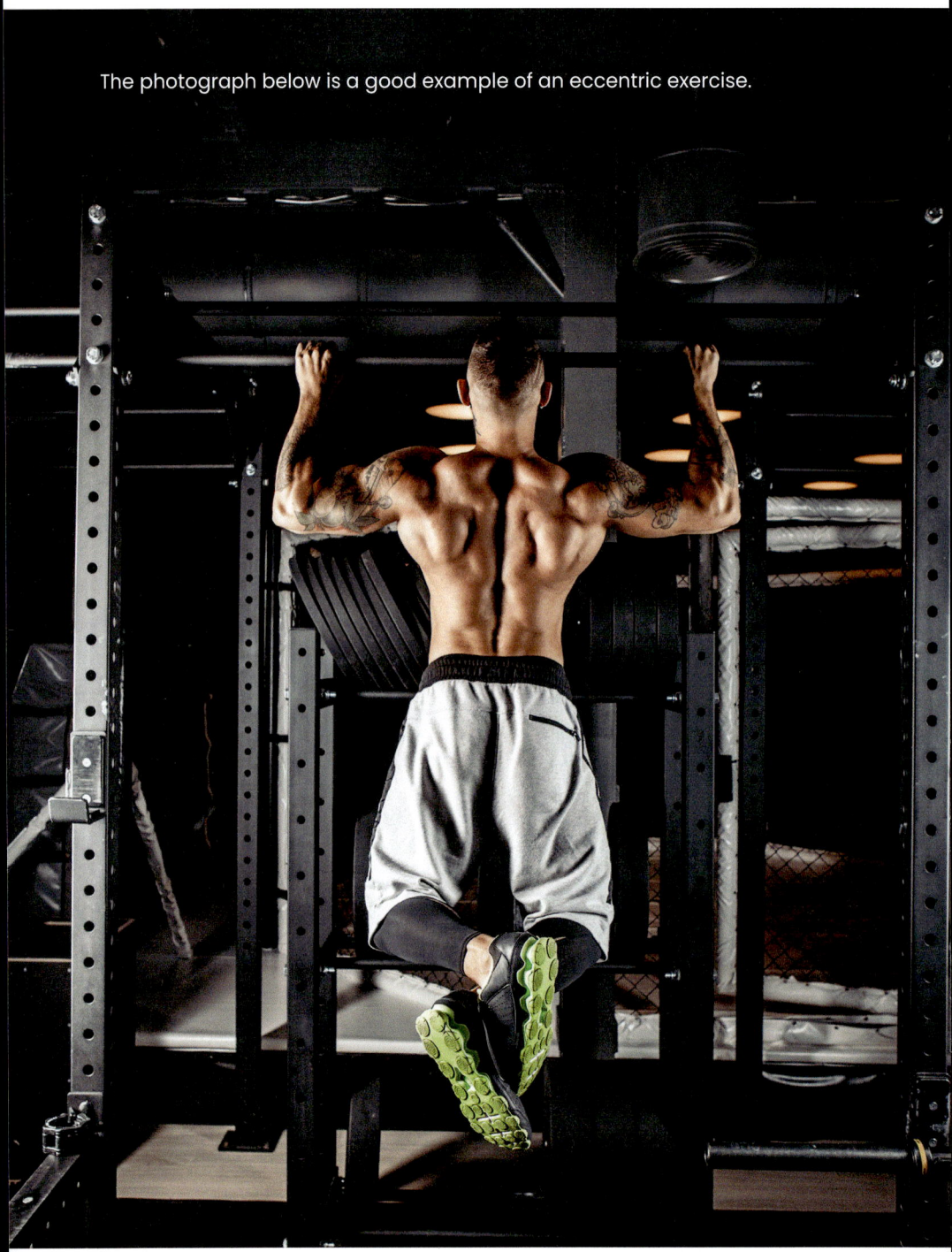

DEVELOPMENT OF MY 100,000 SYSTEM

This exercise is an eccentric pull-up. This sounds misleading as the exercise is about lowering the body slowly, with complete control. The 'eccentric' use of the pulling muscles (upper back and biceps) provides a great addition to **everyone's** training routines.

As with any exercising, the benefit lies in correct administration of these techniques. My 100,000 system incorporates all the best isometric and eccentric exercises.

6. Skeletal/joint/spinal mobility.

It is quite natural and understandable that we don't focus on the things we cannot see – in essence, if we can't see it, we're not interested in it. This certainly seems to be the case with the human skeleton. Look at the image below.

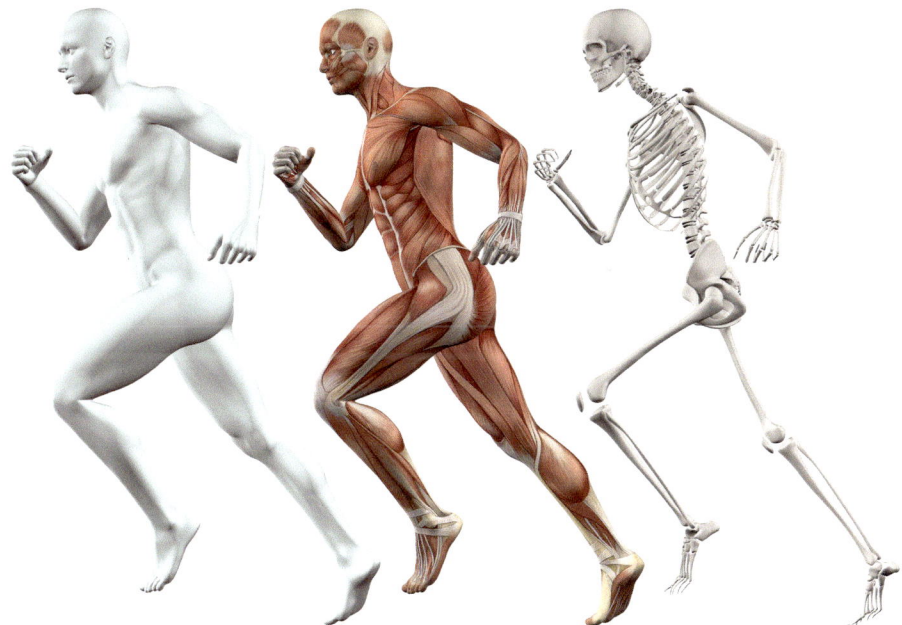

To understand how to exercise the image on the far left, we need to understand the functioning of the middle image (human muscular system) and the far-right image (human skeleton).

As a sport scientist, I have to be acutely aware that all movements, exercises and activities are underpinned by a strong, flexible, mobile and fluid skeleton. All too often a stiff, unresponsive skeletal system provides a great barrier to fluid, co-ordinated exercises and movements.

DEVELOPMENT OF MY 100,000 SYSTEM

This applies to the whole skeleton but specifically to the spine. As I've said, we're all highly individual in our movement patterns – some are flexible, some are not. This is, however, highly trainable, and yet this is another component that seems to be missing in most exercise programmes.

All joints need mobility exercises, but due to its complexity and the enormous stresses and strains that it must endure, it is vital that **you** look after **your** spine. We've seen that the human spine is a remarkable system or structure, capable of amazing things, but the pressures of poor posture, foot mechanics, hip/pelvic mechanics, exercise technique and many other factors put significant demands on and through the spine that must be managed.

I am therefore specifically interested in incorporating skeletal mobility movements into all my programmes. My 100,000 system includes all the necessary exercises that you need, and below is an example of a 'knee roll' movement for lower back (lumbar spine) mobility.

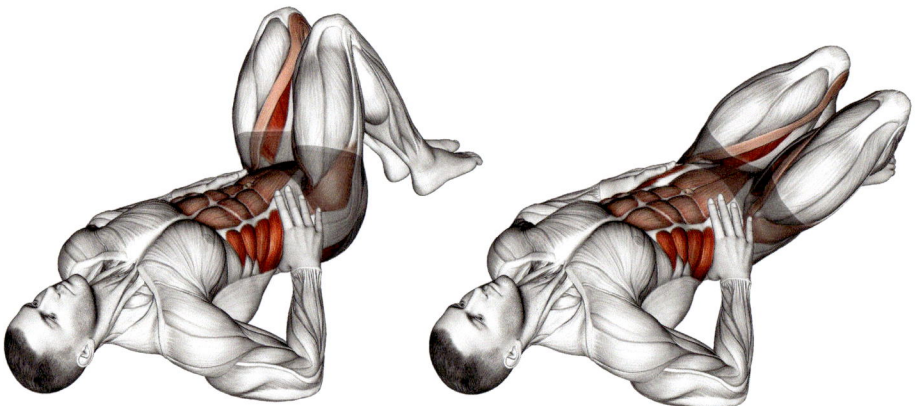

7. Abdominal exercises

The number one request I receive as a sport scientist and personal trainer concerns the perceived need to exercise the abdominal muscles – a 'six-pack' still seems to be the most desired element of all exercisers and exercise programmes. It still seems to be the holy grail. It is probably the most discussed and analysed area of exercise, and yet most individuals are still guessing as to how to train their abdominal muscles correctly.

To begin to understand this complex area, I want to dissect it into three very important components that, as a personal trainer, I must understand to be able to prescribe the correct balance of exercises for each individual.

First, let's consider the anatomy and function of our 'abs'. Below is a diagram of human abdominal muscles (rectus abdominis).

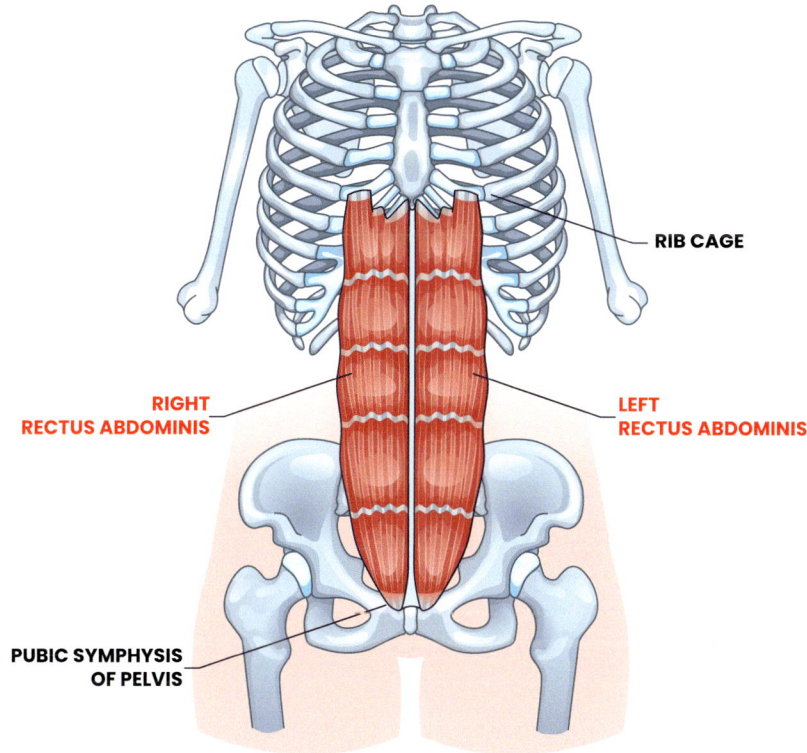

The main functions/actions of the rectus abdominis are:

- Flexion of the trunk (flexion of the thoracic and lumbar spine).
- Tensing the anterior wall of the abdomen.
- Aid in tilting the pelvis.
- Aid core stability.

There exists a battery of exercises to target these all important muscles, from sit-ups, half sit-ups and crunches to reverse, bicycle, oblique, twisted and kick crunches, Russian twists, torso twists, mountain climbers, leg drops, half-leg drops, single leg drops, single leg pulses, scissor kicks, captain's chair, hollow body holds, hanging leg lifts, reach-ups, boat pose and flutter kicks. then there are all the

DEVELOPMENT OF MY 100,000 SYSTEM

various 'miracle' exercises with the many available gadgets. All these exercises are variations that utilise the rectus abdominis muscle function of flexing the trunk (pulling the ribcage forward towards the hips/pelvis).

Second, as I have highlighted, in recent years the whole world has gone core-stability mad. Core stability has become the buzzword for all exercises, but is this correct, and what does it really mean for **you?** As I said above, the rectus abdominis (abdominal muscles) only aids in the stability of the core.

Right is a diagrammatic representation of how the human skeleton 'should' function.

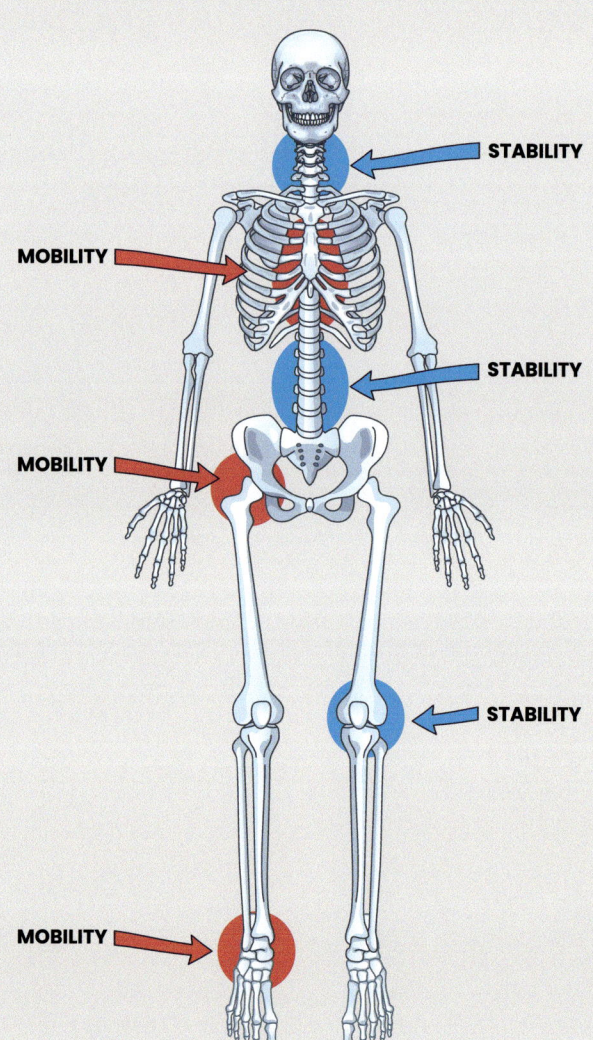

As I explained in previous chapters, the human body is a giant chain, and each link (joint) in the chain must function correctly for the integrity of the whole body to function efficiently. The diagram (right) shows that the cervical spine (neck and shoulders) is designed to provide stability, the thoracic spine (upper and middle back) is built for mobility and the lumbar spine (lower back) is an area for stability. The core of the human body is the area that exists between the ribcage and the hips/pelvis.

DEVELOPMENT OF MY 100,000 SYSTEM

What then is the difference between the abs and the core? The diagram below shows the additional musculature that constitutes the core.

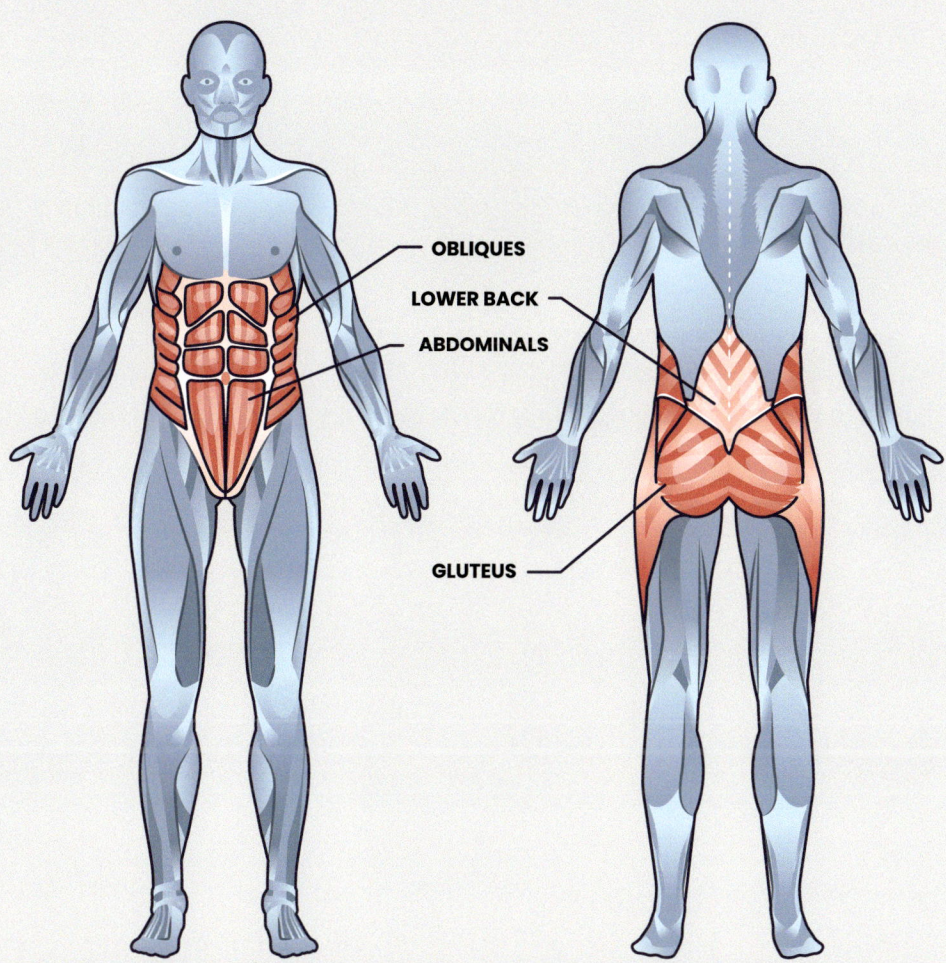

The additional muscles that surround the entire lumbar (lower back) spine – the diaphragm, internal and external obliques, transverse abdominis (TVA), pelvic floor, spinal erectors, quadratus lumborum and multifidus muscles – all play a very significant role in establishing and maintaining the stability of the whole lower spine area. In fact, the rectus abdominis (abdominal) muscle exerts the least amount of stability to this area.

Due to the explosion of interest in the core and the blind belief that it is the be-all and end-all of all exercising, it is my job as a personal trainer to explain and prescribe the correct balance of exercises to meet the needs of each client – to explain and prescribe the correct balance of exercises for **YOU**.

The third area of importance here is the understanding of what exercising these muscles can and cannot achieve. The request I receive most often from clients defining their goals and ambitions is that they want to 'tone up' the whole body, and specifically the abdominal area. Scientifically speaking, the word 'tone' is meaningless, but we all know that the individual means he or she wants to achieve a lean, slim, contoured abdominal area in which the musculature is visible externally.

Let's be abundantly clear here – this lean, slim, contoured look has **absolutely nothing** to do with the rectus abdominis, the TVA or any other muscles. This desired look is not achieved by doing endless crunches or side planks. It's achieved by reducing abdominal subcutaneous (under the skin) fat levels. The diagram below helps to explain this.

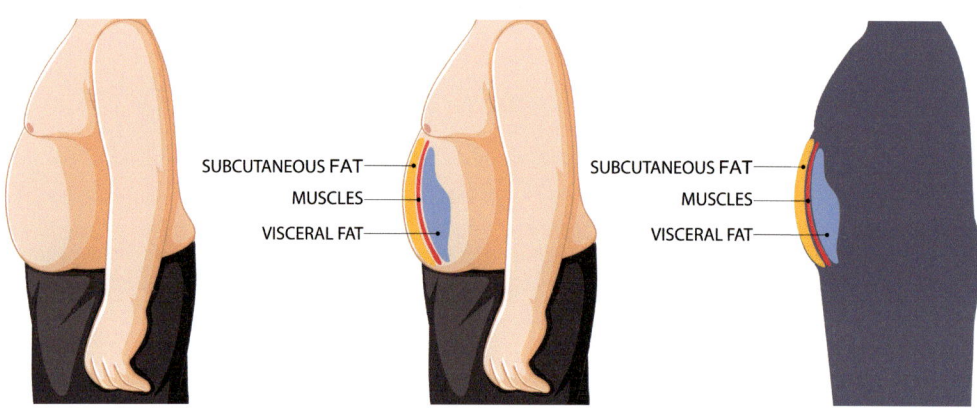

Performing isolation muscle-targeting exercises for the surface and deeper abdominal region **does not** directly 'burn' away the subcutaneous fat that lies between the musculature and the skin surface. So a visual six-pack result will never be attained without addressing the layer of fat that lies above. This is specifically addressed by incorporating many cardio-based exercises into all routines and, of course, attaining very low body-fat levels.

In summary, this highly contentious area of exercising must adopt the perfect balance of traditional abdominal exercises, core-based stability exercises and healthy lifestyle.

I advocate small modifications of the 'traditional' abdominal exercises by incorporating the 'setting of the core' element, which 'sets' the stability to the lower spine allowing for a productive movement that is safe – kind to the spine.

I have worked tirelessly to incorporate the perfect blend of these modified exercises and the more modern core-based movements and positions into my 100,000 system.

As an elite personal trainer, I am always striving to push the boundaries, experiment and develop new ideas, positions, exercises and movements. That said, however, it would be remiss, almost disrespectful, of me to overlook the importance of including many great existing exercises, positions and movements that have been established and practised for decades.

Therefore, my next important challenge in developing my 100,000 system was to discern the good, the bad and the ugly in all other exercise regimes, routines and principles. There are millions of disciples around the world who swear by the benefits of yoga, Pilates, high-intensity interval training (HIIT), speed training, strength training, endurance training, plyometric (dynamic power) training, balance training, myofascial release (foam roller) training and various cardiovascular training techniques.

I am not a fan of simply adopting one exercise principle above all others, and simply do not subscribe to the philosophy that one principle – yoga, for example – can give an individual all the necessary ingredients to achieve their desired result. There is no doubt, however, that there are some very good and important exercises in each and every one of the regimes I've mentioned, and that I needed to incorporate them into my 100,000 routines.

To summarise, the formulation of my 100,000 system has been multifaceted. It has meant cutting out all the rubbish, incorporating new, different and vital components, blending them with the necessary physiotherapy-based musculoskeletal stability exercises and embracing the best current exercises.

Taking into account all of the above, and to ensure that my 100,000 exercise system is the world's most complete, varied and comprehensive regime ever formulated, it needed to be underpinned by 30 vital components that I believe – and indeed have proved – to be vital for each and every one of **you**.

Here is a brief description of each and every one of my vital exercise components. These 30 components are:

DEVELOPMENT OF MY 100,000 SYSTEM

1. Foam roller exercises (myofascial release)

An EVA foam roller was first used in 1987 for self-massage and mobilisation. It is a good and useful gadget, cheap and easy to use and beneficial for increased range of movement, reduced soreness, improved recovery time, relaxation, circulation and decreased stress.

Myofascial tissue is thick connective tissue that spreads in a network throughout your entire body, connecting your muscles, bones and joints. The multi-layered tissue contains liquid called hyaluronan that provides stretch and encourages free range of movement. When this liquid becomes 'sticky' or dries up it can impact on surrounding body parts.

Tight myofascial tissue can restrict movement in your muscles and joints and can lead to widespread pain and discomfort. Applying firm pressure for 30 to 60 seconds to each area can produce and promote great results.

It is a great warm-up exercise and therefore I include it at the top of the list in each and every routine.

2. Dynamic stretching exercises

These increase circulation and blood flow, enhancing agility, speed and muscle strength, making it ideal to include at the start of each workout.

Research has shown that you can improve your sporting performance and help prevent injuries when you include dynamic stretching in your warm-up routines. This is because it activates your nervous system and muscles and improves your joint movement and muscle flexibility as well as your balance and control.

Therefore, dynamic stretching for 30 to 60 seconds at the start of your workout is highly recommended.

3. Nerve stretching/gliding/flossing exercises

These help to improve nerve movement through the joints and muscles by improving their ability to slide and glide. This is very important as so many individuals have underlying nerve tightness.

Nerve pain can cause numbness, tingling, weakness and radiating, moving and referred (different location) pain. Inflammation or adhesions anywhere along the nerve can cause the nerve to have limited mobility and get stuck.

Nerve gliding exercises should not be painful, reaching an intensity level of four or five out of ten.

The major nerve complaint relates to the sciatic nerve. The symptoms of sciatica can vary from mild ache to excruciating pain that radiates along the pathway of your sciatic nerve, which runs from your lower back down through your hips and into each leg. There are symptoms of numbness, tingling or muscle weakness that travel down the back of your thigh and into your lower leg or foot.

Obesity, diabetes, age, a sedentary lifestyle, bone spurs, herniated disks and age-related degeneration can all contribute to joint dysfunction, which may lead to sciatic pain. Sciatica can require significant treatment including drugs, and it can be a lengthy process to recovery. Prevention is therefore crucial and should be included in each and every training programme.

4. Skeletal mobility exercises

These covers the range of uninhibited motion around a joint and are essential for flexibility and fluidity of human movement

As an elite personal trainer, I always work from the inside out, considering the individual's skeleton as an absolute priority. Skeletal mobility movements have been non-existent in most training schedules in the last 30 years, so I insist on these movements in each training session.

They allow you to improve strength, performance and decrease your injury risk during every one of your workouts.

If you look after your skeleton, it will repay you in kind. I have smothered my 100,000 exercise system with my favourite skeletal mobility movements, which I have used with all my clients over many decades.

5. Muscle activation exercises

If you want to get better results and lower your risk of injury, you must include activation exercises at the start of your workouts. These exercises target specific muscles to increase blood flow and activate, or 'wake up', muscle groups.

A good set of activation exercises can prepare your body for the more intense exercises that will follow in your workout. They establish a stronger communication link between your brain and the rest of your body, preparing your body for what's to come. They can reduce the risk of injury significantly and help to relax overactive muscles. The targeted muscles work more effectively so you won't overcompensate with other muscles.

All activation exercises should be low-impact and low-intensity.

6. Pilates and yoga exercises

Specific movements from both disciplines can enhance any exercise programme.

Pilates is a system of exercises to improve physical strength, flexibility and posture and enhance mental awareness. It consists of a series of exercises primarily designed to target the core muscles of your abdominals, hips, glutes, lower back and inner thighs.

Chances are you know someone who does Pilates. It was initially created for dancers to help their overuse injuries by strengthening their core musculature – the muscles that you don't usually use in your day-to-day life. It can also improve body awareness and mindfulness.

Yoga is a spiritual and ascetic discipline that includes breathing control, meditation and adoption of specific bodily postures. It moves the body into various positions to increase flexibility and balance and improve breathing and relaxation.

It has both physical and mental benefits and is often prescribed for the treatment of back pain and arthritis. It is also beneficial for increased energy, alertness, increased muscle strength, weight reduction, maintaining a balanced metabolism and injury prevention.

7. Transverse abdominis (core/TVA) exercises

The TVA is a muscular layer of the anterior and lateral (front and side) abdominal wall. It is a 'corset' muscle, so when it contracts it pulls inwards rather than flexing your trunk forward.

The TVA maintains normal abdominal wall tension and increased intra-abdominal pressure, which helps to support internal organs and viscera and aids expulsive forces such as forced expiration, late stages of childbirth, urination and defecation. It plays a role in almost all movement, so TVA strength can help support your spine and surrounding muscles from injury and help to improve pelvic floor muscles and posture.

Core stability exercises have become a modern-day phenomenon, but most exercisers do not perform these exercises correctly or effectively. I have included only the best TVA positions and movements in all my 100,000 routines.

8. Cardiovascular/cardiorespiratory exercises

These affect the ability of your heart, lungs and blood vessels to transport blood around the body to the working muscles. No matter your age, weight or athletic ability, cardiovascular activity is an absolute must – indeed, most health benefits through adaptations to exercise result from cardiovascular exercise.

During aerobic activity you repeatedly move the muscles in your legs, hips and arms while breathing faster and more deeply, thus maximising the amount of oxygen in your bloodstream. Your heart beats faster, which increases blood flow to your muscles and back to your lungs. Your body will release endorphins, your natural painkillers and mood-enhancing chemicals, promoting a great sense of well-being.

Cardiovascular/cardiorespiratory exercise can increase your metabolic rate, aid in fat loss and increase your stamina, fitness and strength. It can ward off viral illness and significantly reduce heart disease, high blood pressure, diabetes, obesity, resting heart rate, metabolic syndrome, strokes and certain cancers.

It can also manage conditions like arthritis and blood sugar imbalance, directly strengthen your heart muscle and increase its efficiency, keep your arteries clean, boost your HDL (good) cholesterol and lower your LDL (bad) cholesterol, boost your mood, decrease depression, anxiety and tension, increase relaxation, mental health, self-esteem and improve sleep quality.

What's more, it can increase your cognitive function, increasing mental sharpness, judgement, memory and vitality. Cardiovascular exercise is key every time you train.

9. Strength training exercises

Concentric (muscle-shortening) exercises entail the exertion of force on a physical object.

DEVELOPMENT OF MY 100,000 SYSTEM

Also known as weight training, resistance training and/or muscular training, strength training should be a priority for every individual irrespective of age, weight or athletic ability. Muscular hypertrophy results from neuromuscular adaptations from strength training, which can bulletproof your whole musculoskeletal system.

Please here remember my non-negotiable rules: **close your eyes – focus, find, feel and fatigue**. Remember also the importance of **not** counting reps.

10. Balance exercises

Balance in biomechanics is an ability to maintain the line of gravity of a body within the base of support, with minimal postural sway.

Balance training has been an ever-missing component in almost all past and present exercise regimes. Overlooked and underrated, it provides many benefits, strengthens your core, stabilises musculature, helps to prevent injury, cements and promotes brain and body connections and increases posture.

Balance training promotes neuromuscular coordination – the collaboration between your brain and your muscles. Your balance uses the different systems of your eyes (the visual system), which helps you orientate in space, and your inner ear (vestibular system), which records rotary movements and accelerations.

The receptors in your muscles and joints and the pressure receptors in your skin (the proprioceptive system) pass on information to help your posture. These systems work with lightning speed with your brain as a constant feedback loop, to adapt as we coordinate movement.

Balance training improves these important motor skills. It mainly exercises the deep muscles of the trunk and spine, thereby increasing the structural and postural strength of the spine. It's another very important missing link.

11. Gluteal muscle exercises

The 'glutes' are a pelvic muscle group consisting of the gluteus maximus, gluteus medius and gluteus minimus. These muscles are the foundations on which the spinal column sits and link the lower body to the upper, controlling ground reaction forces like shock absorbers.

Historically, the gluteal muscles have been the poor relations among the more glamorous-seeming, 'aesthetic' muscles of the biceps, triceps, shoulders, chest, abdominals and thighs. It may sound ridiculous but, because we can't see them directly, just like the hamstrings, we have much less interest in them.

They have therefore not been a fashionable muscle group over recent decades, and even though the tide is gradually changing, the vitally important glutes, individually and collectively, are still not a priority muscle group.

Biomechanically speaking, the glutes are arguably the human body's most important muscle group and I have always given them priority in my workouts and insisted that training them forms part of every routine. They keep us upright and are responsible for proper pelvic alignment and function, standing (posture), walking, jogging, running, skipping, twisting, arching and bending forwards; sideways and backward propulsion are all the domain of the glutes. Unsurprisingly, they are crucial for lower-back care above and knee function below.

Poor glute function is at pandemic proportions. They really must be star performers and function optimally. That's why they are my number one muscle group in importance, and I include only the best gluteal exercise in all my routines.

12. Back/spinal care exercises

As I said earlier, the whole world is full of back pain, so increasing the strength, flexibility and efficiency of movement of the whole spine is central to the health, fitness, flexibility and condition of the whole body.

Despite the spine being the top source of pain for so many individuals, specific spinal exercises have been completely overlooked for decades in all the exercise regimes we have followed. The resurgence of yoga and Pilates over the last 20 years has tempered the problem, but back pain remains the number one issue for the whole world.

We must learn to look after our skeleton – bones, joints and especially the spine functioning optimally allows the whole body to function beautifully. Targeted spinal/back-care exercises are therefore essential in all training programmes.

13. Hip and pelvis stability exercises

Consisting of the sacrum, coccyx, ischium, ilium, sacroiliac joints and pubis, the hips and pelvis are the hub of the human body, the real unsung heroes of balance, stability, power and shock absorbency.

There are 36 muscles whose sole function is to provide stability, not movement. They're not 'glamorous' muscles, which explains why so many professionals don't understand their importance, position, location or function and hence why crucial exercises remain unprescribed.

They are another vital missing link.

The human body's ability to maintain a neutral pelvic position, providing great body stability during exercise and sports, is essential, so correct targeted exercises for these areas are non-negotiable.

14. Rotator cuff exercises

The rotator cuff muscles (supraspinatus, infraspinatus, teres minor and subscapularis) are a group of muscles that surround the shoulder joint. Individually they all have an important function for the shoulder joint, but their work collectively is crucial.

The rotator cuff muscles work to ensure that the upper arm (humerus) is correctly positioned in the joint socket. If it's not centred correctly, significant stress is placed on the surrounding tissue and cartilage, making the shoulder susceptible to injury.

The human shoulder joint is magnificently unique in that its range of movement is 360 degrees, which makes it incredibly versatile but also quite vulnerable if all the intricate cogs in this slick but very small wheel are not all functioning optimally. Ageing, poor posture, poor upper-spine mobility, recurring lifting and overhead motions, swimming, baseball, tennis and weightlifting all add extra mechanical stress to this joint.

What does this mean for every one of us? It means that anyone who does press-ups, planks, chest presses, chest flies, upright rows, face pulls, pull-ups, chins, shoulder presses, lateral raises, bicep curls, tricep pushdowns, tricep dips, boxing, badminton, squash, basketball and so on ad infinitum simply **must** exercise their rotator cuff muscles correctly and regularly to prevent a host of shoulder issues.

It really is inconceivable to me, as a sport scientist, that anyone should partake in almost any activity, exercise or sport without exercising the rotator cuff musculature.

15. Speed training exercises

These concern the ability to move limbs quickly, using fast-twitch muscle fibres.

As exercise has evolved through the recent boom years, there has been an increasing amount of guidance towards slow, concentrated isolation exercises. Slow, precise, considered technique has become the norm as personal trainers study their clients' movements and technique minutely. While this has great merit, speed exercises have faded into the background.

Our muscles are populated by both fast- and slow-twitch muscle fibres and slow, isolation and endurance training only serve the slow-twitch fibres. This clearly misses out on the significant benefits that can be gained from fast-twitch muscle (speed) training.

Scientific research has concluded that ageing (from 25 years onwards) takes a greater toll on our fast-twitch muscle fibres than on our slow-twitch fibres. In addition, there is an assumption that speed training is somehow more dangerous, making us more vulnerable and more likely to cause ourselves injuries.

This is simply not true. In fact, there are many added benefits to be gained from correct speed work – increased agility, increased anaerobic endurance, increased fat burning, increased muscle, increased power, decreased injury risk, increased balance and proprioception and stronger bones and connective tissue.

It would be criminal to deny your body any one of these extra benefits, so I have included speed training in every workout.

16. Proprioception exercises

Inexplicably, proprioception is a word that very few people, even professionals, have even heard of.

Proprioception, also known as kinaesthesia, is the ability to sense and freely move your body and limbs in your external environment (spatial awareness). It involves a close relationship between the nervous system, soft tissue and proprioceptors. Proprioceptors are specialised sensors located on nerve endings in your muscles, tendons, joints, skin and inner ear; these sensors feed back information about changes in position, movement, force, tension and environment to your brain.

Proprioception is crucial in all sports, exercise and fitness activities. Proprioception training can reduce your risk of injury, increase your balance and increase reaction times, coordination and agility.

The vestibular (spatial orientation) system, vision (eyesight) and proprioception systems all send signals to your brain to sort and integrate sensory information. Your brain then transmits signals to the muscles that are responsible for movement, to help maintain balance and vision of the environment.

I have developed key proprioception training exercises that you **must** incorporate into your training.

17. Eccentric muscle contraction exercises

As we've seen, muscle strength training consists of three key phases – the concentric, isometric and eccentric phases. The lifting, shortening, positive phase is the concentric portion of the movement; the stationary, static or transition point is the isometric phase; and the lowering, lengthening or negative phase is the eccentric contraction – the motion of an active muscle that is lengthening under load.

During eccentric contractions, the external force of the weight and/or gravity is greater than the force you generate to move it – hence why it is referred to as 'negative' reps. Eccentric muscle strength is necessary for everyday life and specifically beneficial for stability, mobility and injury prevention. Eccentric work can cause delayed onset muscular soreness (DOMS) and neural adaptations.

Importantly, metabolically speaking, eccentric contractions require about one quarter of the energy of concentric contractions and produce more muscle force. Therefore the input-reward ratio is highly favourable for eccentric work compared to traditional concentric work, which in turn can lead to greater muscle hypertrophy (growth).

Highly beneficial for injury protection, eccentric muscle work has been seriously overlooked but **must** now be seen as a vital component of modern training.

18. Postural training exercises

Our posture, defined as the position assumed by the body because of the coordinated actions performed by a group of muscles working to maintain stability, has significant consequences for our overall health.

Poor posture due to tight or weak muscles, stress, obesity, wearing unsupportive shoes, poor stance and the use of computers and mobile phones can lead to breathing problems, headaches, poor mood and significant back pain. On the other hand, good posture can have a profound effect on our health and wellbeing.

Proper alignment of our bones and joints has significant effects on our body's biomechanical capabilities. Posture is an automatic and unconscious position, and it represents the body's reaction to the force of gravity.

Proprioceptive maturation of the foot at around five or six years of age establishes the three physiological curves that balance the spine (dorsal kyphosis, cervical and lumbar lordosis). As discussed previously, 'tech neck' – the forward head position adopted in response to the use especially of mobile phones – is becoming the next biomechanical pandemic.

The exercising world has been too busy striving for weight loss and aesthetic muscle shaping to spend any time working on vital postural exercises. They are vital positions, movements and exercises, essential for the maintenance of postural alignment, flexibility and structural strength, and should be deep rooted in all exercise programmes.

19. Sacroiliac joint stability exercises

Forming part of the hips and pelvis, as discussed above in component 13, the sacroiliac joints deserve their own special attention.

During my 37 years' experience I have very rarely come across individuals or trainers who understand the anatomy and biomechanical influence of the SI joints. Testing, stretching and exercising these joints is another vital missing link in all past and present exercise philosophies. Sacroiliac dysfunction and pain are commonplace, and this is a check that I perform with every one of my clients.

Hypermobile Ehlers-Danlos (EDS) syndrome is an inherited genetic disorder caused by gene mutations that affects connective tissue, ligaments and cartilage. The SI joints are one of the strongest joints in the body but EDS and other causes – injury, arthritis, pregnancy and infection – can cause SI dysfunction, which can result in many symptoms in the buttocks and groin but with the main result being lower-back pain.

Sacroiliac joint stability exercises **must** be considered essential as they provide great stability during all complex body movements. They are another missing link and hence a vital component of all routines.

20. Compound movement exercises

As with speed training, compound exercises have gone out of fashion somewhat during the age of isolation exercising, but they can play a vital role in our health and fitness.

Compound movements and exercises engage multiple muscle groups and joints at the same time and provide a myriad of additional benefits – building more muscle mass and strength, improving mobility and muscular balance, increasing calorie consumption and reducing the risk of injury.

Please don't shy away from compound movements just because they're tough. Let's remember the benefits and the importance of these powerful, muscle-building movements. They complement all other exercises beautifully.

21. Abdominal exercises

The number one request from my clients relates to the abdominal area of the body – the obsessive pursuit of a flat stomach dominates most individuals' exercise goals.

Traditional abdominal exercises and a very gradual realisation that a few crunches won't flatten your stomach have given way to the new world obsession of core stability. I have already discussed core stability in some detail, but it must be highlighted that there should not be a fight between the two.

The traditional abdominals (rectus abdominis) form part of the body's core, and exercises targeting both sets of musculature complement each other. Good abdominal muscle strength aids breathing, prevents lower back pain, stabilises the spine, aids posture and provides the strength and balance needed for almost all exercises, movements and activities, allowing athletes to transfer more energy from their core to their limbs and increasing performance. And the added benefit of a visual six-pack is a very welcome side effect of good abdominal work.

Don't let the traditional abdominal exercises fade away. Provided that you follow my golden rule of *focus, find, feel and fatigue* and hence perform the exercises correctly, good abdominals are a must.

22. Iliotibial band exercises

The iliotibial band is a thick band of fascia, composed of dense fibrous connective tissue, that runs down the lateral side of the thigh. Its function is to help extend, abduct and rotate the hip; it also helps to stabilise the knee joint and is very important in lower extremity motion.

It is also a common location for injury. Iliotibial band syndrome presents pain and/or tenderness on palpation of the lateral aspect of the knee, superior to the joint line and inferior to the lateral femoral epicondyle. Often referred to as runner's knee, it is particularly vulnerable to overuse of repetitive movements and concomitant with underlying weakness of the hip adductor muscles.

Thankfully, there has been an increase in awareness of IT band importance in recent years, however the established trend of treating it is **completely** wrong; I discussed this in more detail earlier on.

Suffice it to say the commonplace occurrence of IT band syndrome warrants much greater attention from every one of us, irrespective of our training objectives. I have therefore included stretches, positions, movements and exercises specifically to target this important and problematic area.

23. Knee stability exercises

Second only to back pain, knee joint pain in its many forms is so commonplace and debilitating that it must be a main priority for almost every exerciser.

The stability of the knee joint is dependent on dynamic and static factors. The main static stabilisers are the ligaments (medial collateral, lateral collateral, anterior and posterior cruciate ligaments), while the dynamic stabilisers are all the surrounding muscles. The combined influence of the muscles and the ligaments determines knee joint stability during positions, movements and exercises, but the emphasis lies in the strengthening of the dynamic stabilisers (muscles).

As the knee joint is so integral to overall human biomechanics, it must be given the attention it requires and I therefore include many dedicated knee pre- and rehabilitation exercises in my 100,000 programmes that are non-negotiable.

24. Isometric muscle training exercises

As stated in component 17, isometric contraction of muscles occurs with no visible movement of the joint. Even though isometric contractions are the poor relation of muscular work, they

DEVELOPMENT OF MY 100,000 SYSTEM

have been proved to help joint stability, build muscle strength, balance and range of movement, reduce stress, improve mental health and help in injury prevention.

There are two types of isometric contraction exercises – those that we hold statically (isometrically) and those that we push isometrically. Isometric muscle work therefore deserves its place in my 30 components in its own right, but as I have said repeatedly, variety and complementary components produce much greater results. So in conjunction with traditional concentric muscle exercise and the important inclusion of eccentric exercises, isometric muscle work is a great addition to any workout.

25. Plyometric training exercises

Plyometric exercises combine strength training and cardiovascular exercise in each movement. The 'killing two birds with one stone' principle of exercise with plyometrics seems to have had its time in the limelight – the use of plyometrics has been controversial at times and it has been reduced to the status of an old-fashioned exercise philosophy.

While one could argue for a slightly greater injury risk, well-executed plyometric exercise can seriously enhance anyone's training. Plyometrics help you jump higher, run faster, lift heavier and develop more power. They can build strength, increase your speed and power, burn body fat and improve overall muscle definition by training your anaerobic system and cardiovascular system together.

This mode of training, which can also improve coordination and agility, can benefit every individual and is a great additional component of any exercise programme.

26. Swiss ball exercises

The Swiss ball is a great modern addition to the exercising family. It provides variety and versatility and can be incorporated into both warm-up and warm-down procedures, Pilates, yoga, resistance training, flexibility work and general gym work – and, of course, it has become synonymous with core stability exercises.

Just sitting on a Swiss ball engages the key stabilisers: the abdominal and back muscles. The balance element involved forces you to support your own weight and stabilise yourself. It is great for balance and proprioception exercises and for many posterior chain muscle exercises.

The Swiss ball is another brilliant addition to my 30 key components.

DEVELOPMENT OF MY 100,000 SYSTEM

27. Ankle joint stability exercises

I have addressed the phenomenal importance of human biomechanics to our overall exercising strategy and stressed the significance of skeletal joint stability. The foot/ankle stability issue is therefore right at the front of the queue – foot contact with the floor and hence ankle mechanics initiate the highly critical kinetic chain of motion that radiates up through the entire body.

I've shown how essential it is to establish efficiency throughout this chain, through **every** muscle and joint, but of course, each segment can only act and react to the efficiency, position and movement of the previous segment.

If this kinetic chain starts poorly or inefficiently, the rest of the chain has no chance; it will just initiate a series of compensatory patterns that would ravage even the most robust skeletal system.

Foot/ankle stability exercises are therefore imperative in all exercise programmes.

28. Muscular endurance exercise

This is the ability of a muscle to remain active over a long period of time, using slow-twitch muscle fibres.

Historically and traditionally isolated muscle strengthening exercises are geared to using moderate or, most often, heavy weights to fatigue a muscle over a short period of time. While this still predominates for strength gains, the use of light or lighter weights, pushing the muscle to fatigue with a much greater number of repetitions, must **not** be overlooked.

As I've explained, one of my non-negotiable rules is: do *not* count your repetitions, learn to 'tune in' to your muscles and judge each and every set of exercises on the feeling, not simply the number of reps.

That said, however, I always incorporate a 100-repetition muscle endurance component into every one of my routines. One hundred reps sounds extreme and, in fact, that is exactly why it works – there should be a number of repetitions that is almost unreachable or unachievable, allowing for a short pause and rest during the set in trying to conquer this endurance challenge. The set produces not only great fatigue but also a feeling of great depth to the exercise. It also not only provides added variety, it also allows time to focus, find, feel and fatigue – explore muscles in great depth.

DEVELOPMENT OF MY 100,000 SYSTEM

You may frequently feel that you can fatigue your muscles to a much greater degree with muscular endurance techniques, not simply relying on traditional strength training exercises. Understanding that muscle fatigue is the key to muscle growth, strength and development ensures that endurance muscular work is high on the list of importance for your overall muscular conditioning.

Other benefits include increased metabolism, decreased fatigue, improved posture, decreased injury, increased back stability due to the endurance of the trunk muscles and increased sporting performance.

Endurance exercise has been a missing ingredient for decades and I strongly advocate its use every time you train. Learn to banish the myth that you cannot increase your strength with muscular endurance exercises.

29. Elastic exercise band exercises

Another great addition to the exercising family, exercise bands provide great variety and versatility and allow for many exercises to be performed in varying planes of movement, not relying on the effects of gravity for muscular resistance. Initially only used in the physiotherapy rehabilitation field, elastic bands are easy to use and provide a great addition to traditional training.

They can really improve your quality of exercise as they encourage greater focus on the movement. Having complete control over how you are using the band, set-up position, angle and movement, you need to be really focused on the feel of each exercise.

There is also a greater 'negative' phase to each movement as you control the band back to the starting position, thereby maintaining greater muscle force throughout the entire movement.

These bands, which come in all sorts of sizes and levels of resistance, are good for many pre- and rehabilitation exercises of the smaller, intricate muscles of the shoulders, wrists and ankles, and equally great for many big compound movements like pull-ups and chins.

Lightweight and highly versatile, they must be included in modern exercise routines.

30. Static stretching exercises

Even though there have been differing opinions over the value, benefit and usage of stretching, it is generally accepted that stretching muscles can only be beneficial for overall muscle and joint range of movement, flexibility and subtleness.

What has been misunderstood is exactly how to perform these stretches. Should they be dynamic or static? How long should we perform them? When should we do them?

Traditionally, 30-second static stretches employed at the start, warm-up phase of exercising have been the norm, but this is **not** correct. Static stretching exercises in preparation for dynamic exercising do not make sense logically and scientifically and can even be counterproductive, decreasing performance and even increasing the risk of injury.

Static stretching, however, has fundamental positive effects on muscles and joints. The foundations of many philosophies of exercise such as yoga, static stretches have untold benefit on overall physical and mental wellbeing and **must** be included. Therapeutic static muscle stretching or rehabilitation can often be up to three minutes, but I strongly recommend at least one minute per stretch per muscle.

It is imperative to realise that static stretching should be performed at the end of each of your workouts and in-between your workout sessions or days.

Summary

In summary: each one of these components is vital for each and every one of you, whatever your age, height, weight, goals or level of experience.

The last 40 years have kicked up methodologies that have mainly focused on a core of just two, three or four elements – they are either strength, cardio, stretching, isolation or compound exercise regimes that are limited in their diversity and one-dimensional in their approach. One-dimensional routines produce, at best, one-dimensional results.

The benefit of these components individually is substantial, but the real magic happens when they are all used each and every time you exercise so that their combined benefit is substantially greater than the sum of the individual parts.

Flooding your exercise routines with positions, stretches, movements and exercises that comfort and soothe your body while having focused intensity produces dramatic results. They can banish hamstring tightness, free up your feet and ankles, stabilise your knees, reassure your hips and pelvis, rid your body of low level and/or acute back pain and promote a stronger, more flexible spine, which in turn promotes better posture, which in turn releases your body from pain and allows it to flourish like never before.

As I blended these 30 vital components into 30 ongoing exercise routines encompassing the exercise norms of warming up, warming down, strength training, variations of intensity and diversity, all in perfect ratio, blend and balance of large versus small muscle groups, upper and lower body exercises, isolation and compound exercises, heavy and light weight, high reps and low reps, it all became quite a jigsaw puzzle – a hugely detailed exercise 'spreadsheet' totalling 900 exercises all working in perfect harmony with each other, as shown (right) and in more detail on the following pages.

The foundations of these programmes are built around the strength training element – major muscle groups following the traditional push/pull philosophy of chest exercises followed by tricep exercises, back exercises followed by bicep exercises, with leg exercises coupled together with shoulder exercises and extra

SUMMARY

abdominal exercises, forming a six-day cycle.

This muscle group cycle is then complemented by the other components, each focusing on the same primary muscle groups for that routine. For example, the strength training muscle group or segment – ie the chest muscle group – is complemented and supplemented by all the other associated chest positions, stretches and conditioning exercises for flexibility and function.

This intrinsic blend of 900 exercises has been tried and tested repeatedly with thousands of clients over many decades.

The detailed, comprehensive 'spreadsheet' of exercises looks very complex in its written form. The reality is that it is unbelievably simple.

For you it just means 30 exercises every time you train. Some of these exercises take only 30 seconds while others may take ten minutes, so if you follow my advice on how to exercise by using my *focus, find, feel and fatigue* mantra, you have a perfectly delivered routine in 40 to 45 minutes that can change your body and your life.

The unique quality of these programmes is that they can be put down and picked up freely. Scientific research dictates that, unlike the 30-minute, three-times-a-week training schedules of the 1980s, we now know that a much greater regularity and frequency of exercising is necessary for maximum exercise progression.

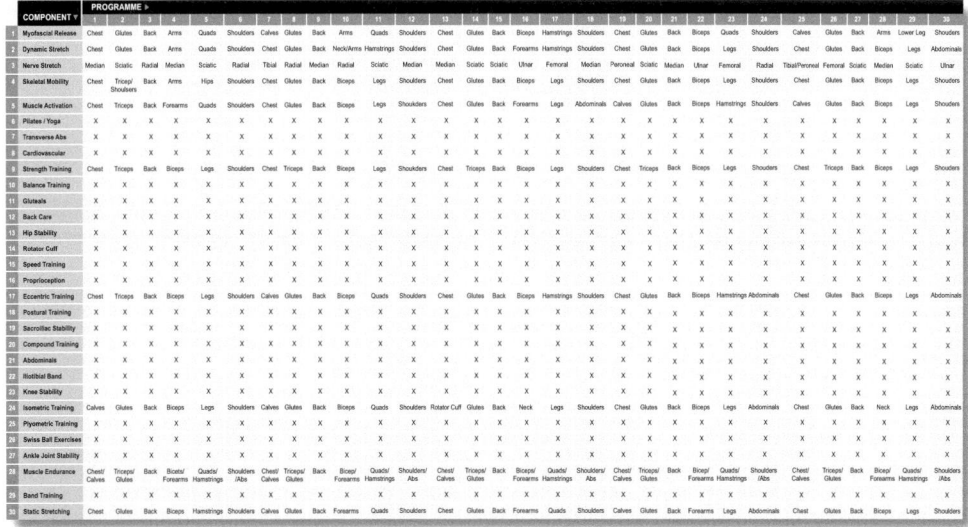

SUMMARY

	COMPONENT	PROGRAMME 1	2	3	4	5	6	7	8	9	10	11	12	13
1	Myofascial Release	Chest	Glutes	Back	Arms	Quads	Shoulders	Calves	Glutes	Back	Arms	Quads	Shoulders	Chest	Gl
2	Dynamic Stretch	Chest	Glutes	Back	Arms	Quads	Shoulders	Chest	Glutes	Back	Neck/Arms	Hamstrings	Shoulders	Chest	Gl
3	Nerve Stretch	Median	Sciatic	Radial	Median	Sciatic	Radial	Tibial	Radial	Median	Radial	Sciatic	Median	Median	Sc
4	Skeletal Mobility	Chest	Tricep/Shoulsers	Back	Arms	Hips	Shoulders	Chest	Glutes	Back	Biceps	Legs	Shoulders	Chest	Gl
5	Muscle Activation	Chest	Triceps	Back	Forearms	Quads	Shoulders	Chest	Glutes	Back	Biceps	Legs	Shoukders	Chest	Gl
6	Pilates / Yoga	X	X	X	X	X	X	X	X	X	X	X	X	X	
7	Transverse Abs	X	X	X	X	X	X	X	X	X	X	X	X	X	
8	Cardiovascular	X	X	X	X	X	X	X	X	X	X	X	X	X	
9	Strength Training	Chest	Triceps	Back	Biceps	Legs	Shoulders	Chest	Triceps	Back	Biceps	Legs	Shoukders	Chest	Tri
10	Balance Training	X	X	X	X	X	X	X	X	X	X	X	X	X	
11	Gluteals	X	X	X	X	X	X	X	X	X	X	X	X	X	
12	Back Care	X	X	X	X	X	X	X	X	X	X	X	X	X	
13	Hip Stability	X	X	X	X	X	X	X	X	X	X	X	X	X	
14	Rotator Cuff	X	X	X	X	X	X	X	X	X	X	X	X	X	
15	Speed Training	X	X	X	X	X	X	X	X	X	X	X	X	X	
16	Proprioception	X	X	X	X	X	X	X	X	X	X	X	X	X	
17	Eccentric Training	Chest	Triceps	Back	Biceps	Legs	Shoulders	Calves	Glutes	Back	Biceps	Quads	Shoulders	Chest	Gl
18	Postural Training	X	X	X	X	X	X	X	X	X	X	X	X	X	
19	Sacroiliac Stability	X	X	X	X	X	X	X	X	X	X	X	X	X	
20	Compound Training	X	X	X	X	X	X	X	X	X	X	X	X	X	
21	Abdominals	X	X	X	X	X	X	X	X	X	X	X	X	X	
22	Iliotibial Band	X	X	X	X	X	X	X	X	X	X	X	X	X	
23	Knee Stability	X	X	X	X	X	X	X	X	X	X	X	X	X	
24	Isometric Training	Calves	Glutes	Back	Biceps	Legs	Shoulders	Calves	Glutes	Back	Biceps	Quads	Shoulders	Rotator Cuff	Gl
25	Plyometric Training	X	X	X	X	X	X	X	X	X	X	X	X	X	
26	Swiss Ball Exercises	X	X	X	X	X	X	X	X	X	X	X	X	X	
27	Ankle Joint Stability	X	X	X	X	X	X	X	X	X	X	X	X	X	
28	Muscle Endurance	Chest/Calves	Triceps/Glutes	Back	Bicets/Forearms	Quads/Hamstrings	Shoulders/Abs	Chest/Calves	Triceps/Glutes	Back	Bicep/Forearms	Quads/Hamstrings	Shoulders/Abs	Chest/Calves	Tri/Gl
29	Band Training	X	X	X	X	X	X	X	X	X	X	X	X	X	
30	Static Stretching	Chest	Glutes	Back	Biceps	Hamstrings	Shoulders	Calves	Glutes	Back	Forearms	Quads	Shoulders	Chest	Gl

SUMMARY

	16	17	18	19	20	21	22	23	24	25	26	27	28	29	30
	Biceps	Hamstrings	Shoulders	Chest	Glutes	Back	Biceps	Quads	Shoulders	Calves	Glutes	Back	Arms	Lower Leg	Shoulders
	Forearms	Hamstrings	Shoulders	Chest	Glutes	Back	Biceps	Legs	Shoulders	Chest	Glutes	Back	Biceps	Legs	Abdominals
	Ulnar	Femoral	Median	Peroneal	Sciatic	Median	Ulnar	Femoral	Radial	Tibial/Peroneal	Femoral	Sciatic	Median	Sciatic	Ulnar
	Biceps	Legs	Shoulders	Chest	Glutes	Back	Biceps	Legs	Shoulders	Chest	Glutes	Back	Biceps	Legs	Shoulders
	Forearms	Legs	Abdominals	Calves	Glutes	Back	Biceps	Hamstrings	Shoulders	Calves	Glutes	Back	Biceps	Legs	Shoulders
	X	X	X	X	X	X	X	X	X	X	X	X	X	X	X
	X	X	X	X	X	X	X	X	X	X	X	X	X	X	X
	X	X	X	X	X	X	X	X	X	X	X	X	X	X	X
	Biceps	Legs	Shoulders	Chest	Triceps	Back	Biceps	Legs	Shoulders	Chest	Triceps	Back	Biceps	Legs	Shoulders
	X	X	X	X	X	X	X	X	X	X	X	X	X	X	X
	X	X	X	X	X	X	X	X	X	X	X	X	X	X	X
	X	X	X	X	X	X	X	X	X	X	X	X	X	X	X
	X	X	X	X	X	X	X	X	X	X	X	X	X	X	X
	X	X	X	X	X	X	X	X	X	X	X	X	X	X	X
	X	X	X	X	X	X	X	X	X	X	X	X	X	X	X
	Biceps	Hamstrings	Shoulders	Chest	Glutes	Back	Biceps	Hamstrings	Abdominals	Chest	Glutes	Back	Biceps	Legs	Abdominals
	X	X	X	X	X	X	X	X	X	X	X	X	X	X	X
	X	X	X	X	X	X	X	X	X	X	X	X	X	X	X
	X	X	X	X	X	X	X	X	X	X	X	X	X	X	X
	X	X	X	X	X	X	X	X	X	X	X	X	X	X	X
	X	X	X	X	X	X	X	X	X	X	X	X	X	X	X
	X	X	X	X	X	X	X	X	X	X	X	X	X	X	X
	Neck	Legs	Shoulders	Chest	Glutes	Back	Biceps	Legs	Abdominals	Chest	Glutes	Back	Neck	Legs	Abdominals
	X	X	X	X	X	X	X	X	X	X	X	X	X	X	X
	X	X	X	X	X	X	X	X	X	X	X	X	X	X	X
	X	X	X	X	X	X	X	X	X	X	X	X	X	X	X
	Biceps/Forearms	Quads/Hamstrings	Shoulders/Abs	Chest/Calves	Triceps/Glutes	Back	Bicep/Forearms	Quads/Hamstrings	Shoulders/Abs	Chest/Calves	Triceps/Glutes	Back	Bicep/Forearms	Quads/Hamstrings	Shoulders/Abs
	X	X	X	X	X	X	X	X	X	X	X	X	X	X	X
	Forearms	Quads	Shoulders	Calves	Glutes	Back	Forearms	Legs	Abdominals	Chest	Glutes	Back	Biceps	Legs	Shoulders

SUMMARY

I always recommend very regular exercise, but let me clarify what this means. In a modern world where everyone's time is at a premium and distractions are all around us, even five to ten minutes most days constitutes regular exercise. In an ideal world, 40 or 50-minute sessions four to six times a week would be the ideal, but this is simply not achievable for everyone, or indeed anyone, each and every week.

Having said that, a realisation that so many individuals *overtrain* has grown. The exercising boom has led to obsession among many, who spend multiple hours every day in the gym. This is simply not necessary – it's even counterproductive and very much not recommended. However dedicated and however driven an individual is to succeed, sheer volume of training is not the answer. One should not train multiple hours in a day and certainly not train seven days a week.

Quality, not quantity is the key.

Please remember that the physiological need for recovery is essential to progress. Exercise, after all, is just the stimulus for change. The changes that we are exercising for are mostly accomplished during this recovery phase from exercise, so resting times and days off are crucial.

Also at this juncture it is prudent to remember that there are **no** miracle exercises or daily routines that can produce miraculous changes in a short period of time. Exercise progress and results are **not** measured exercise by exercise and **not** measured hourly or daily. The transformative, miraculous majesty of responses to exercising is measured by its consistency, week after week.

But what does this mean for you? Over a period of four to six weeks it is important that you complete each and every one of these 900 exercises, but it doesn't mean that you have to complete them in this strict 30 x 30 pattern.

The real magic of these programmes is that they are completely interchangeable. For example, you don't have to perform a dynamic leg/quadricep stretch on the same occasion as your quadricep/squatting exercise day. You don't have to perform your sciatic nerve stretch on the same day as your hamstring training.

Interchanging different exercises with different elements provides an almost unlimited variation in your routines. As I have stressed, *variety* is everything in exercise and my 100,000 system means that you will **never** have to do the same routine twice. It will take care of every aspect of your physical health and fitness and you will see and experience results like never before.

SUMMARY

This is why my 100,000 system is not just a series of exercise routines; it's an education in **you**, an education in exercise and an education for life with exercise routines for life.

Let's look at an example training programme containing each of my 30 vital components.

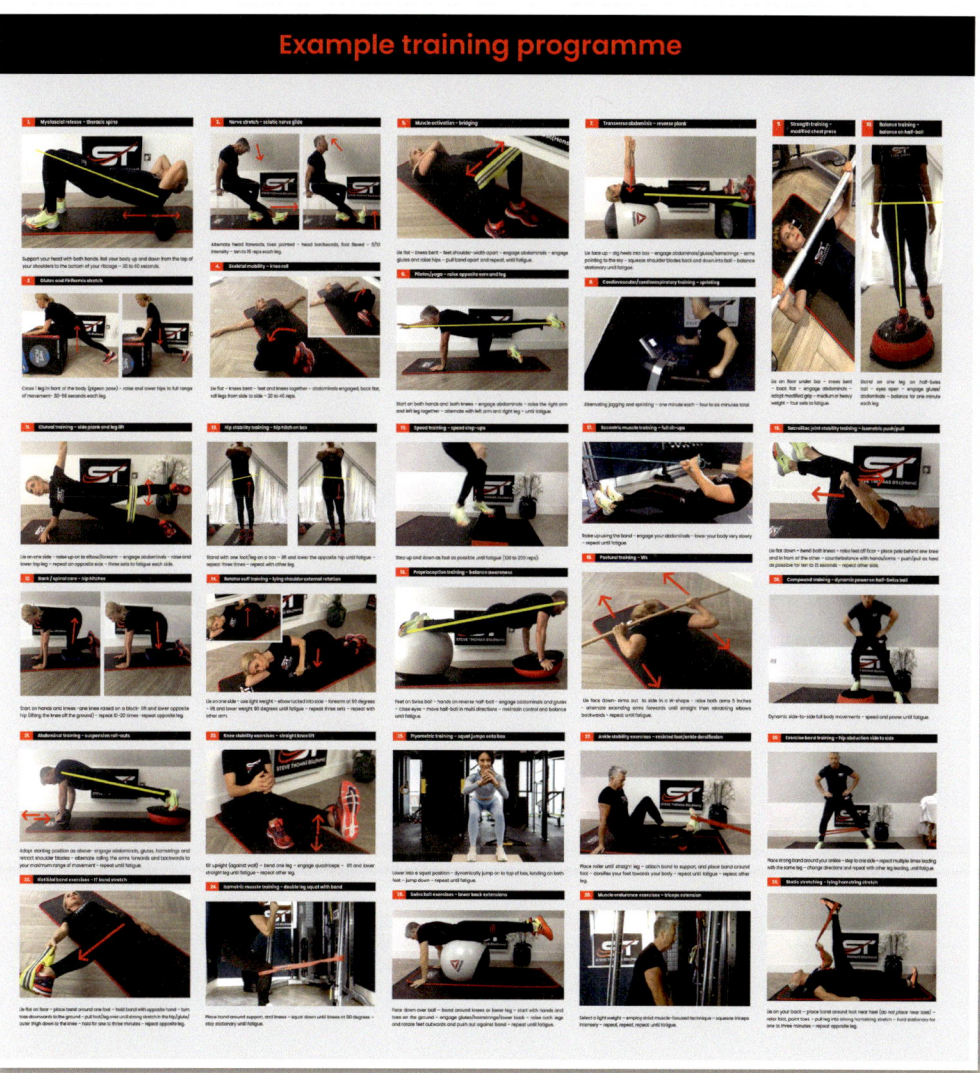

The following section shows the 30 components in easy to follow steps...

SUMMARY

Example training programme

1. Myofascial release – thoracic spine

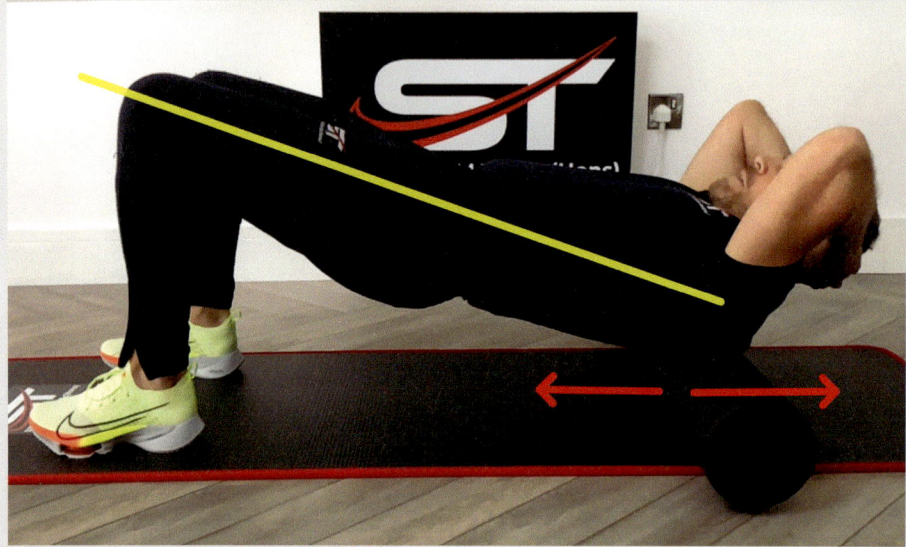

Support your head with both hands. Roll your body up and down from the top of your shoulders to the bottom of your ribcage – 30 to 60 seconds.

2. Dynamic Stretch - glutes and piriformis

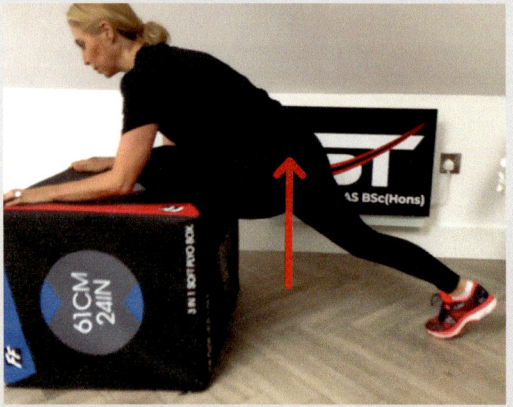 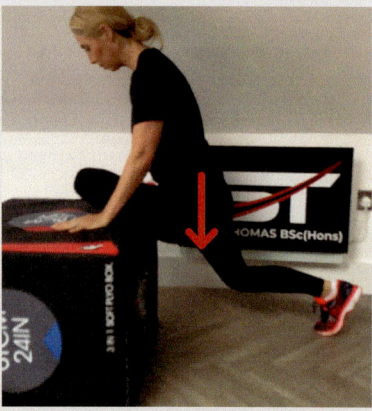

Cross 1 leg in front of the body (pigeon pose) - raise and lower hips to full range of movement- 30-60 seconds each leg.

SUMMARY

3. Nerve stretch – sciatic nerve glide

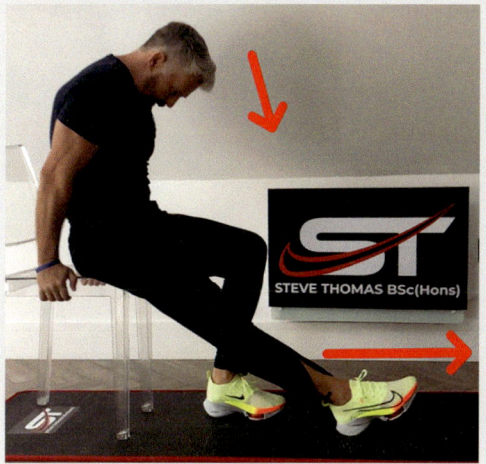
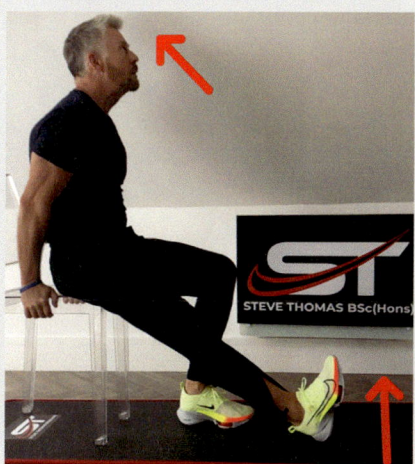

Alternate head forwards, toes pointed – head backwards, foot flexed – 5/10 intensity – ten to 15 reps each leg.

4. Skeletal mobility – knee roll

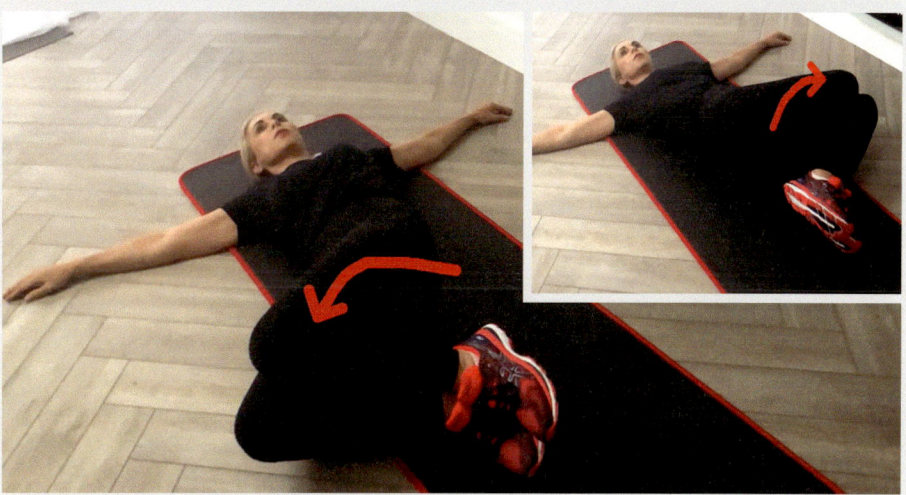

Lie flat – knees bent – feet and knees together – abdominals engaged, back flat, roll legs from side to side – 20 to 40 reps.

SUMMARY

5. Muscle activation – bridging

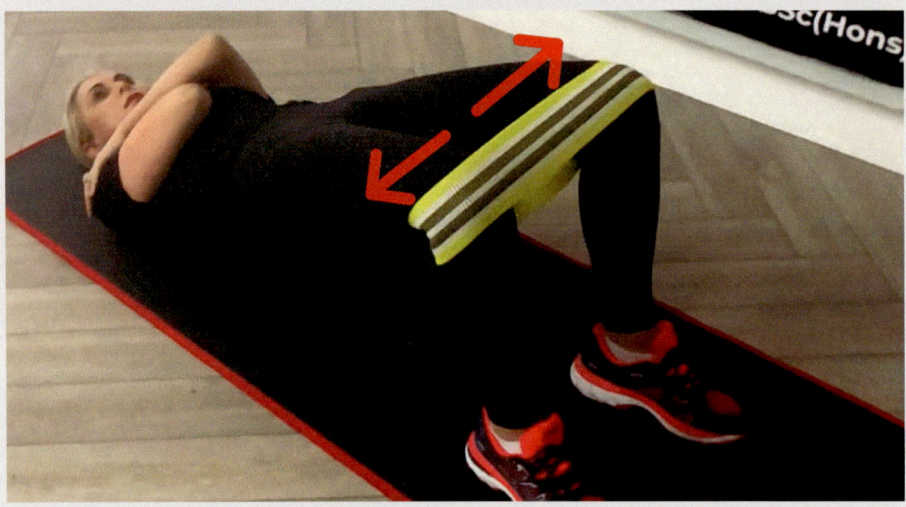

Lie flat – knees bent – feet shoulder-width apart – engage abdominals – engage glutes and raise hips – pull band apart and repeat, until fatigue.

6. Pilates/yoga – raise opposite arm and leg

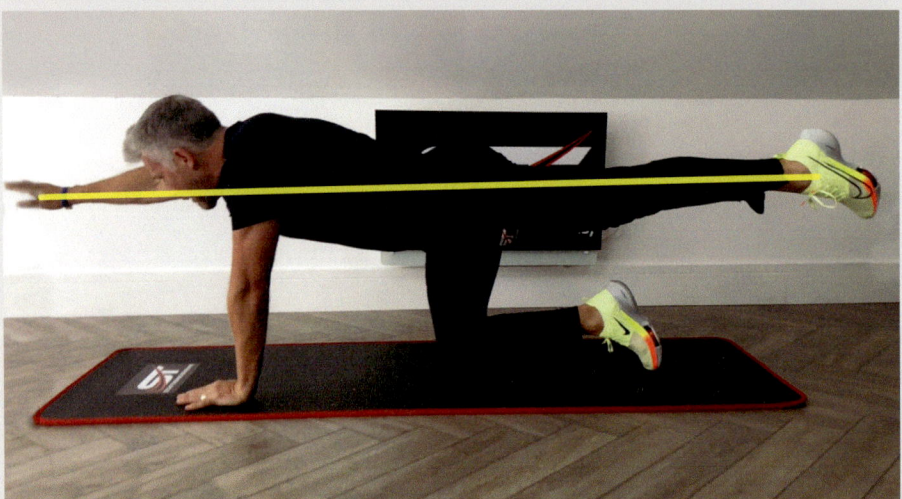

Start on both hands and both knees – engage abdominals – raise the right arm and left leg together – alternate with left arm and right leg – until fatigue.

SUMMARY

7. Transverse abdominis – reverse plank

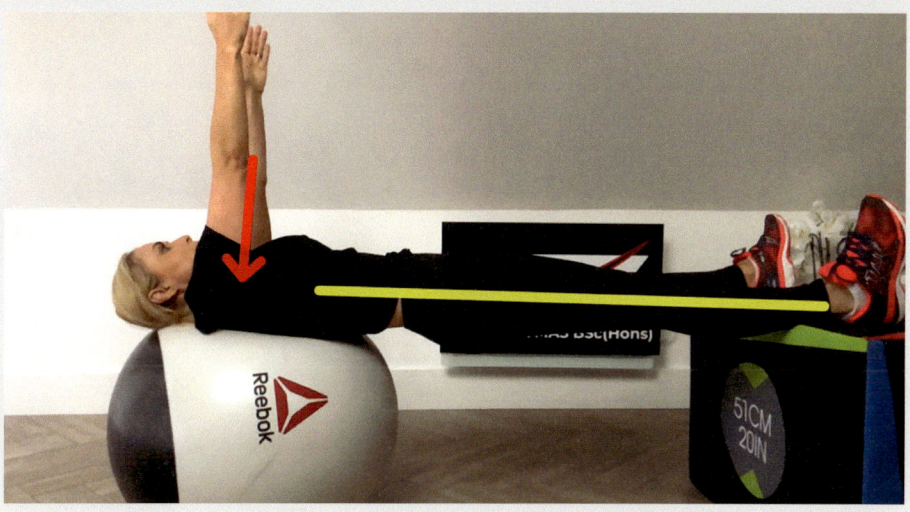

Lie face up – dig heels into box – engage abdominals/glutes/hamstrings – arms pointing to the sky – squeeze shoulder blades back and down into ball – balance stationary until fatigue.

8. Cardiovascular/cardiorespiratory training – sprinting

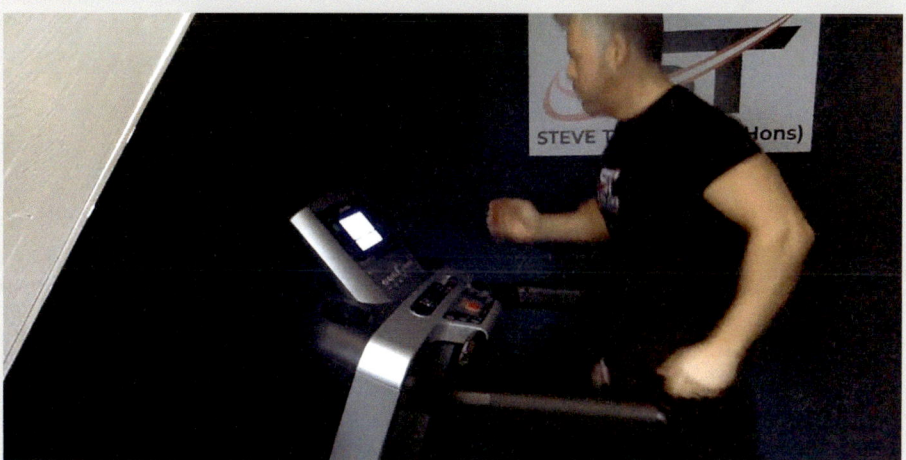

Alternating jogging and sprinting – one minute each – four to six minutes total.

SUMMARY

9. Strength training – modified chest press

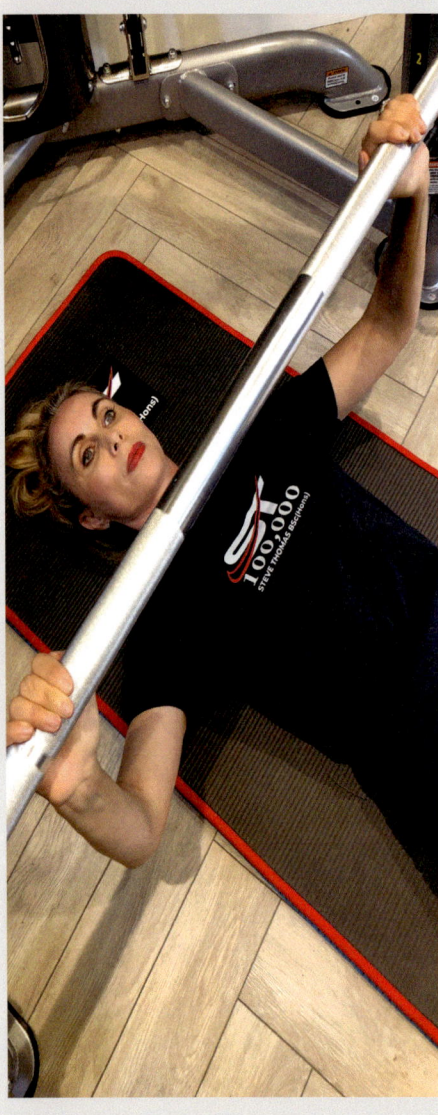

Lie on floor under bar – knees bent – back flat – engage abdominals – adopt modified grip – medium or heavy weight – four sets to fatigue.

10. Balance training – balance on half-ball

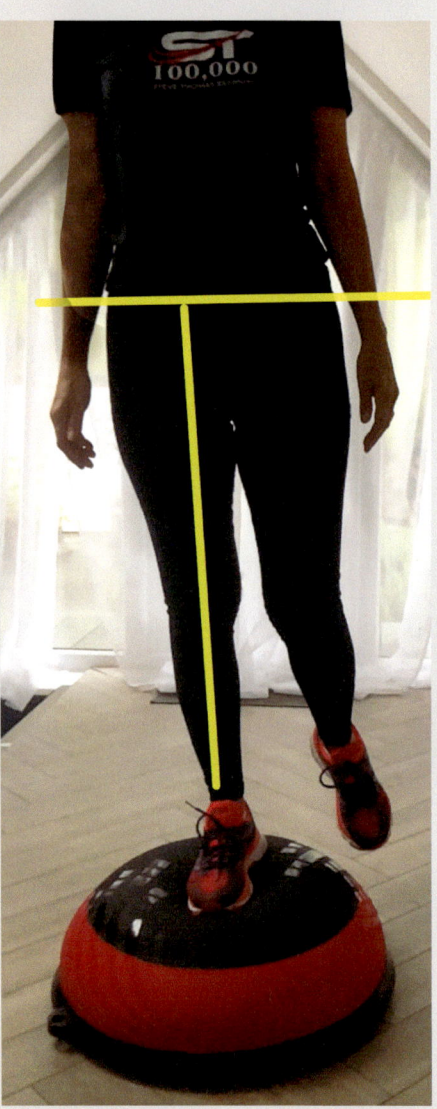

Stand on one leg on half-Swiss ball – eyes open – engage glutes/abdominals – balance for one minute each leg.

SUMMARY

11. Gluteal training – side plank and leg lift

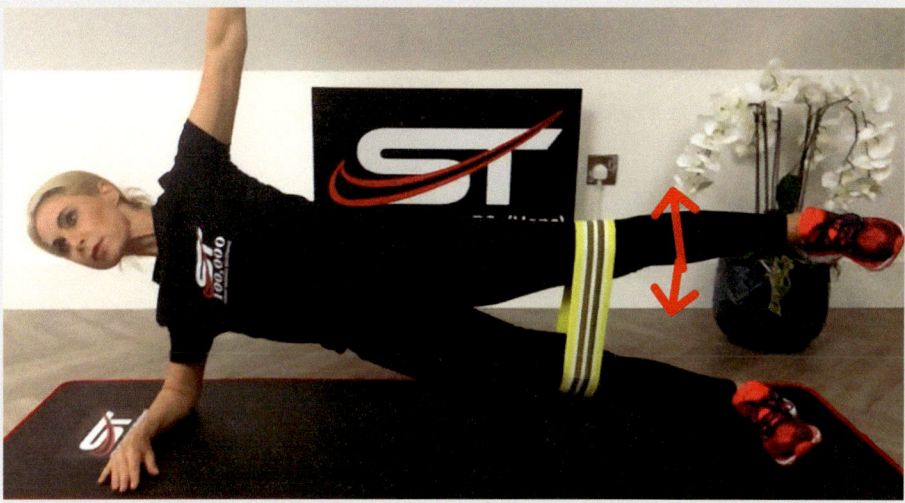

Lie on one side – raise up on to elbow/forearm – engage abdominals – raise and lower top leg – repeat on opposite side – three sets to fatigue each side.

12. Back / spinal care - hip hitches

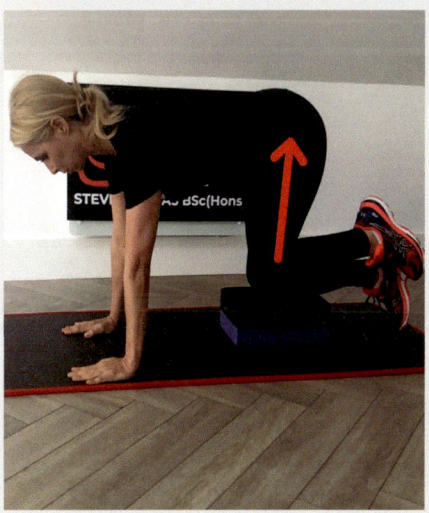 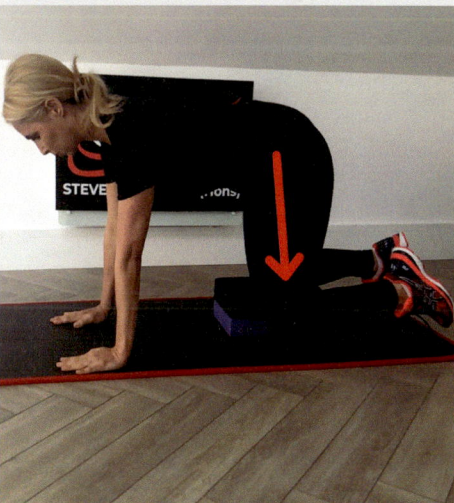

Start on hands and knees - one knee raised on a block- lift and lower opposite hip (lifting the knee off the ground) - repeat 10-20 times -repeat opposite leg.

The FATHER FIGURE of FITNESS

SUMMARY

13. Hip stability training – hip hitch on box

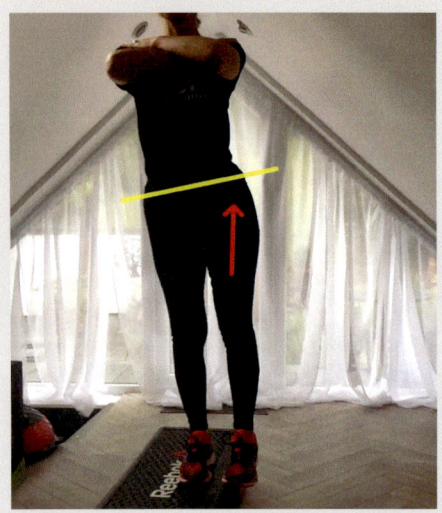
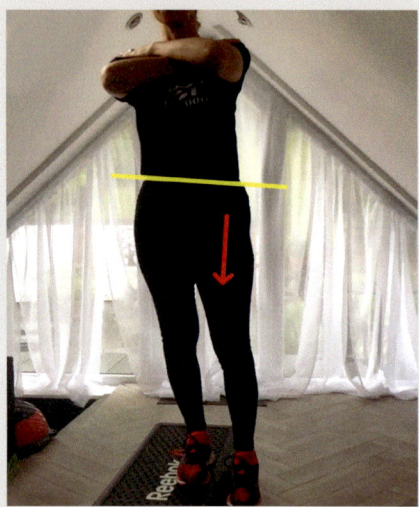

Stand with one foot/leg on a box – lift and lower the opposite hip until fatigue – repeat three times – repeat with other leg.

14. Rotator cuff training – lying shoulder external rotation

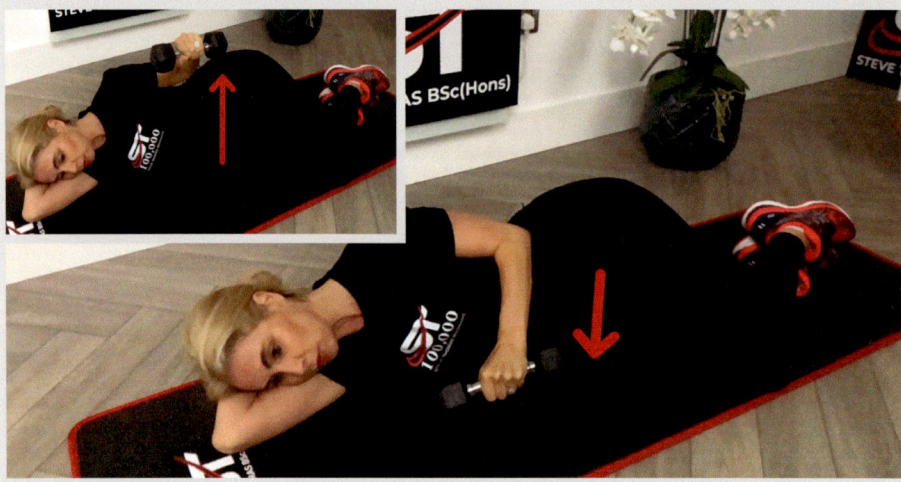

Lie on one side – use light weight – elbow tucked into side – forearm at 90 degrees – lift and lower weight 90 degrees until fatigue – repeat three sets – repeat with other arm.

| 15. | **Speed training – speed step-ups** |

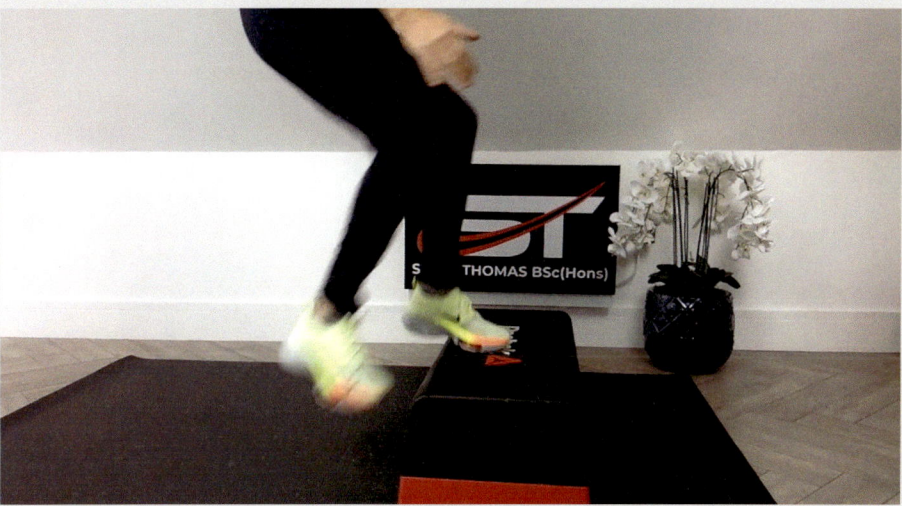

Step up and down as fast as possible until fatigue (100 to 200 reps).

| 16. | **Proprioception training – balance awareness** |

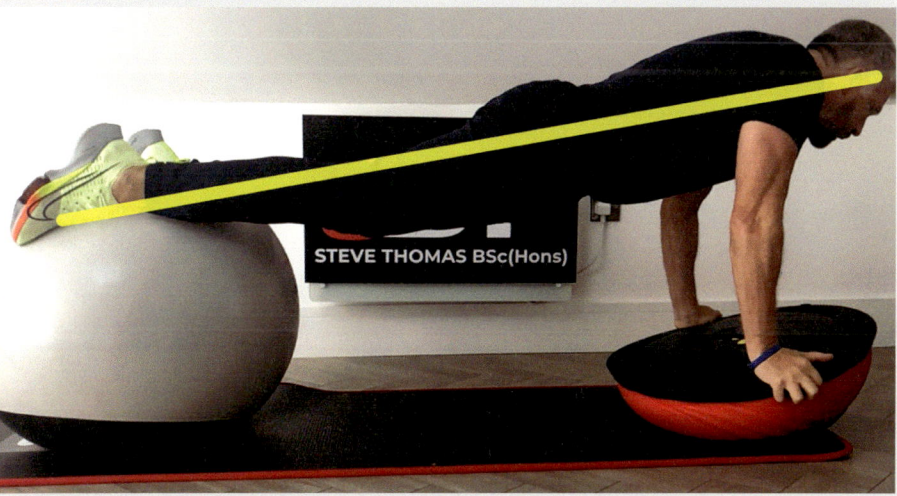

Feet on Swiss ball – hands on reverse half-ball – engage abdominals and glutes – close eyes – move half-ball in multi directions – maintain control and balance until fatigue.

SUMMARY

17. Eccentric muscle training – full sit-ups

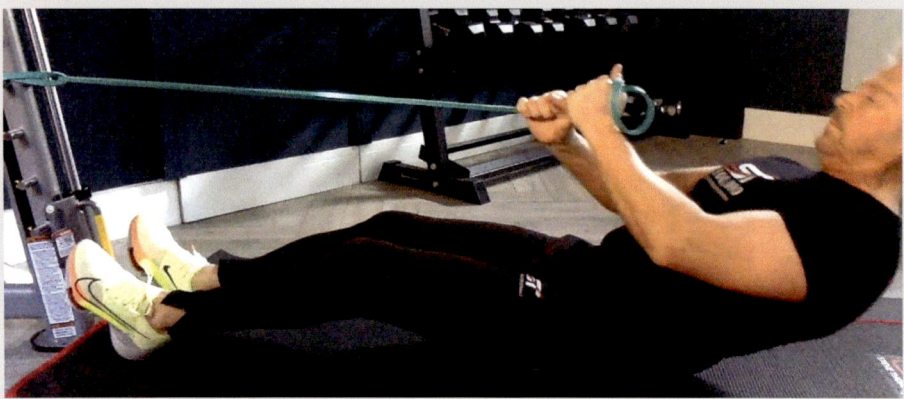

Raise up using the band – engage your abdominals – lower your body very slowly – repeat until fatigue.

18. Postural training – Ws

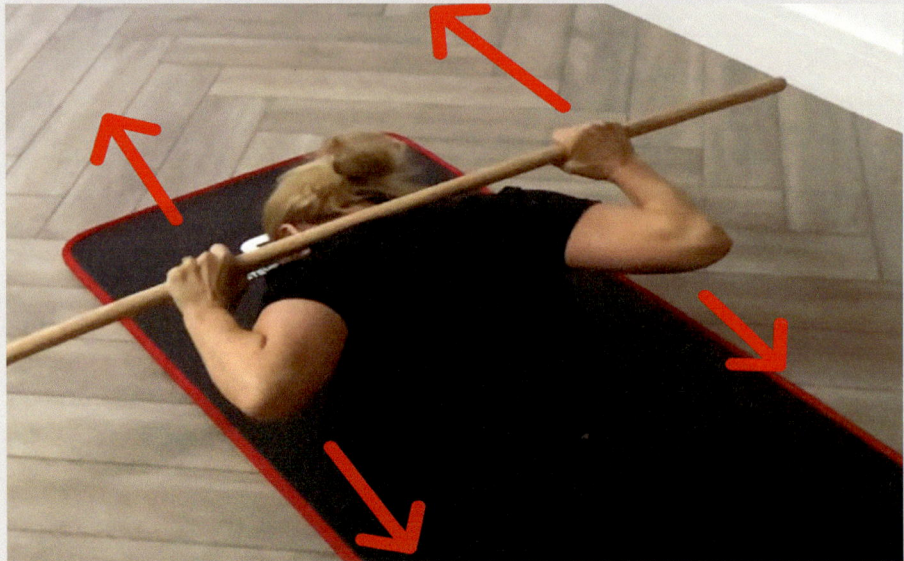

Lie face down- arms out to side in a W-shape - raise both arms 5 inches - alternate extending arms forwards until straight then retracting elbows backwards - repeat until fatigue.

SUMMARY

| 19. | Sacroiliac joint stability training – isometric push/pull |

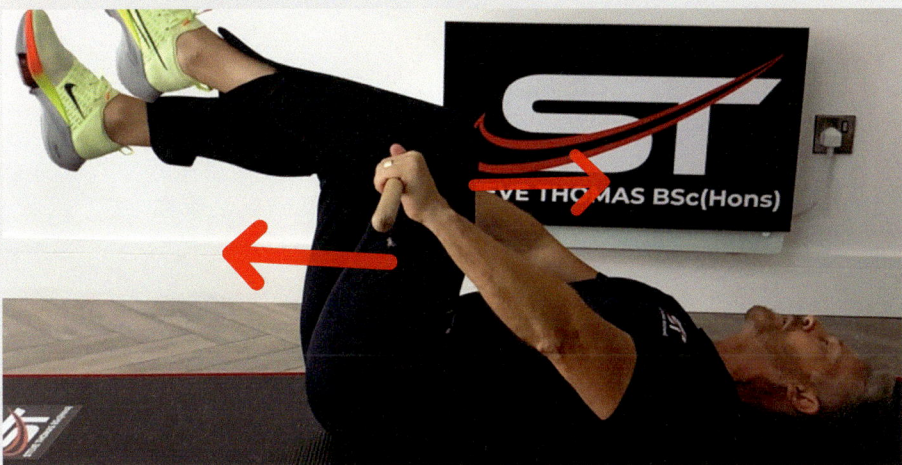

Lie flat down – bend both knees – raise feet off floor – place pole behind one knee and in front of the other – counterbalance with hands/arms – push/pull as hard as possible for ten to 15 seconds – repeat other side.

| 20. | Compound training – dynamic power on half-Swiss ball |

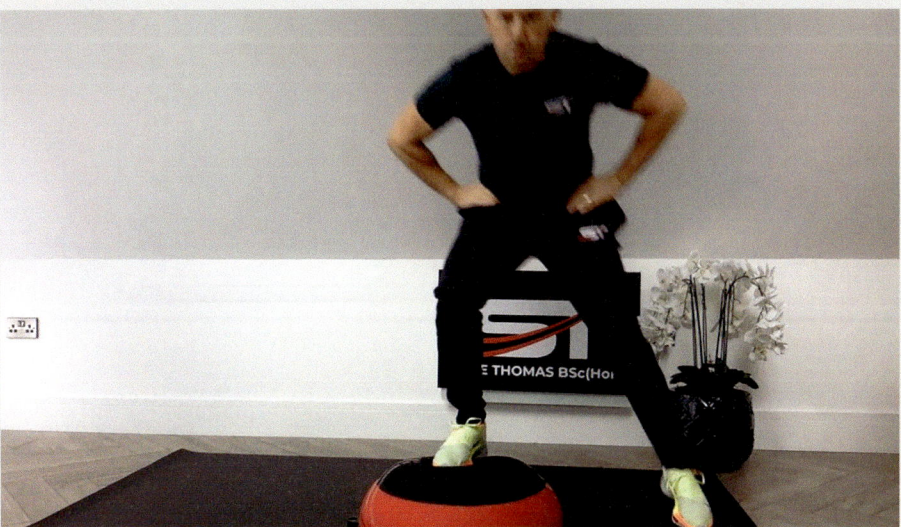

Dynamic side-to-side full body movements – speed and power until fatigue.

SUMMARY

21. Abdominal training - suspension roll-outs

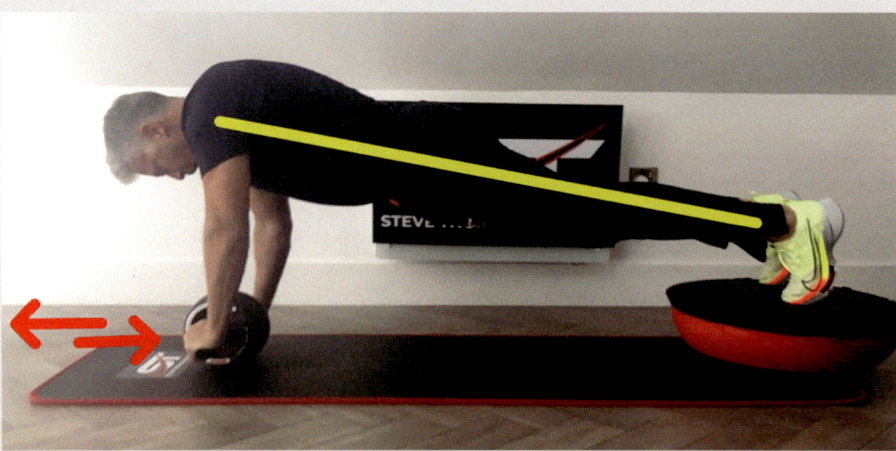

Adopt starting position as above- engage abdominals, glutes, hamstrings and retract shoulder blades - alternate rolling the arms forwards and backwards to your maximum range of movement - repeat until fatigue.

22. Iliotibial band exercises – IT band stretch

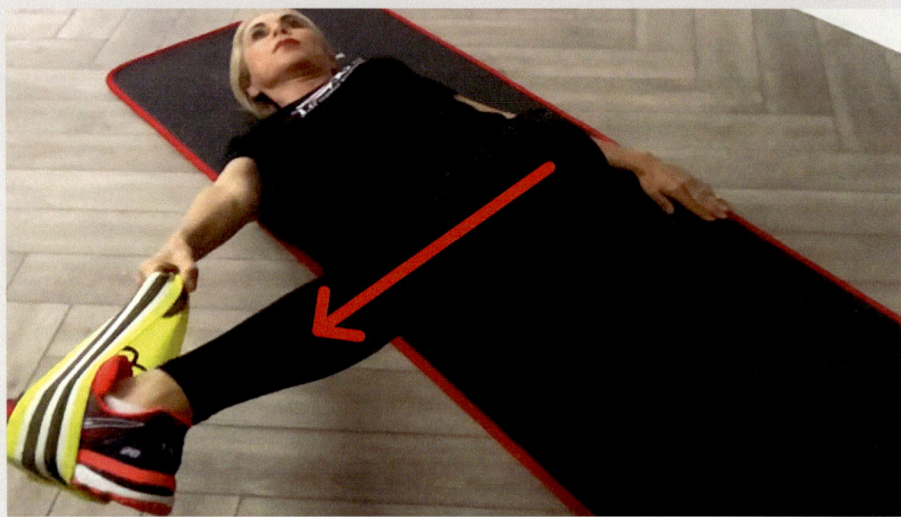

Lie flat on floor – place band around one foot – hold band with opposite hand – turn toes downwards to the ground – pull foot/leg over until strong stretch in the hip/glute/outer thigh down to the knee – hold for one to three minutes – repeat opposite leg.

SUMMARY

23. Knee stability exercises – straight knee lift

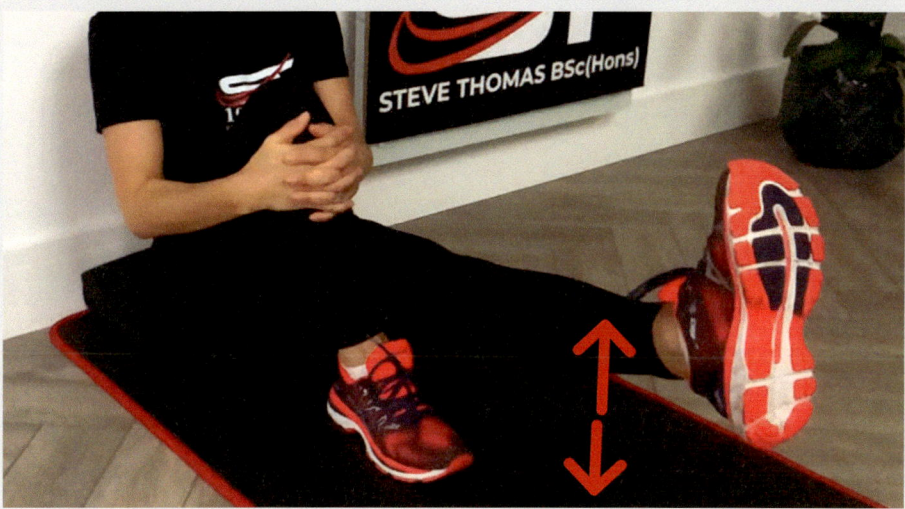

Sit upright (against wall) – bend one leg – engage quadriceps – lift and lower straight leg until fatigue – repeat other leg.

24. Isometric muscle training – double leg squat with band

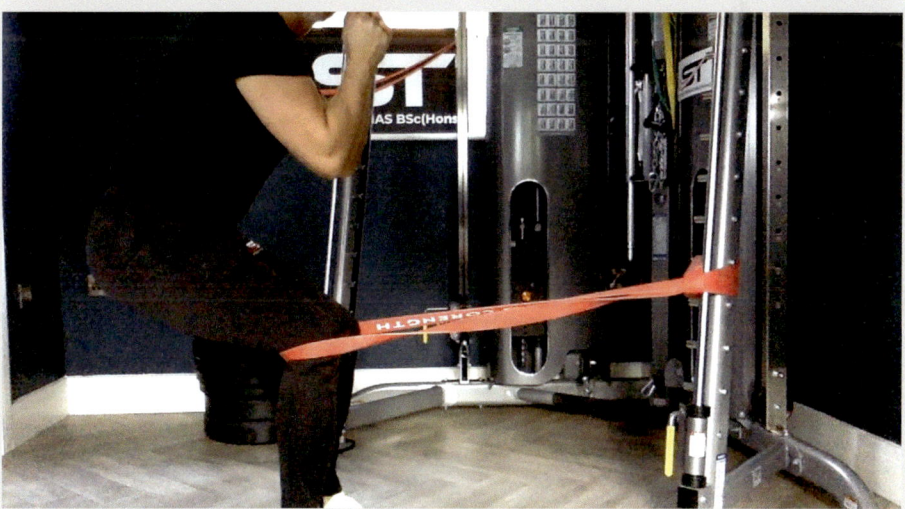

Place band around support, and knees – squat down until knees at 90 degrees – stay stationary until fatigue.

SUMMARY

| 25. | **Plyometric training – squat jumps onto box** |

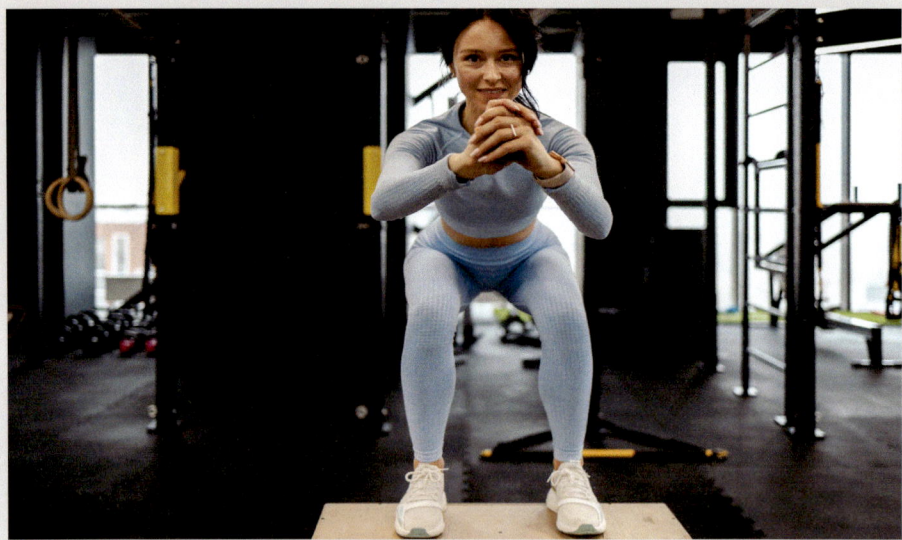

Lower into a squat position – dynamically jump on to top of box, landing on both feet – jump down – repeat until fatigue.

| 26. | **Swiss ball exercises – lower back extensions** |

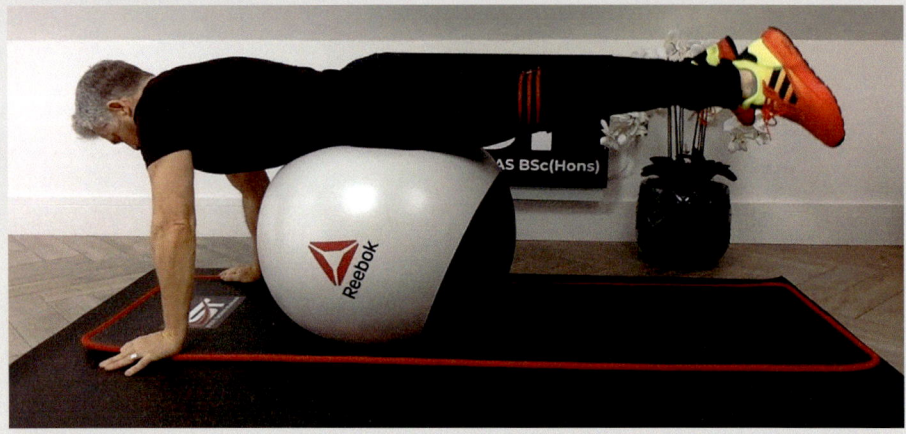

Face down over ball – band around knees or lower leg – start with hands and toes on the ground – engage glutes/hamstrings/lower back – raise both legs and rotate feet outwards and push out against band – repeat until fatigue.

27. Ankle stability exercises – resisted foot/ankle dorsiflexion

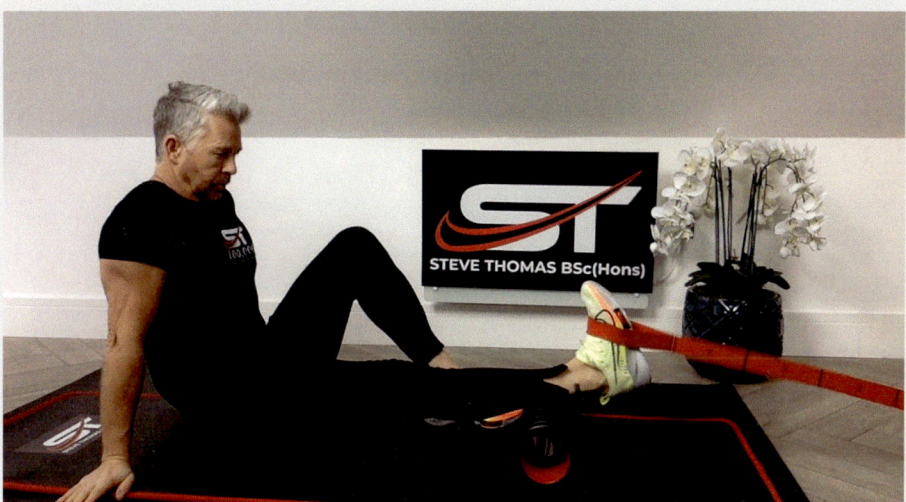

Place roller until straight leg – attach band to support, and place band around foot – dorsiflex your foot towards your body – repeat until fatigue – repeat other leg.

28. Muscle endurance exercises – triceps extension

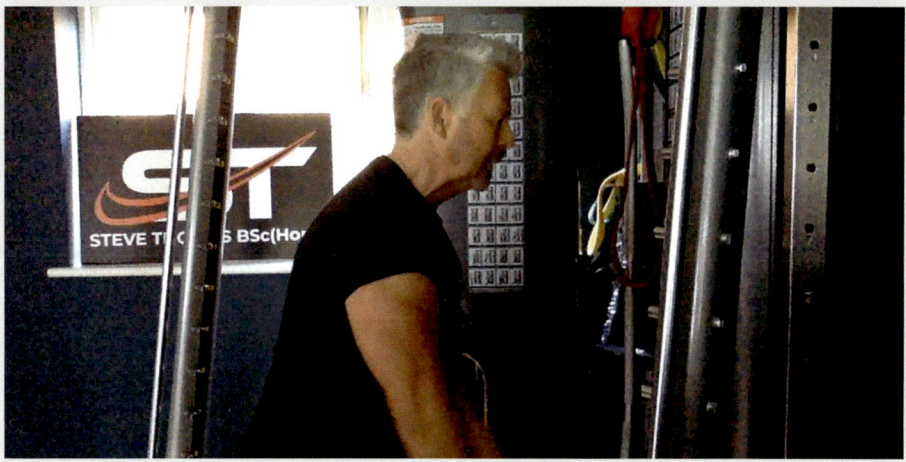

Select a light weight – employ strict muscle-focused technique – squeeze triceps intensely – repeat, repeat, repeat until fatigue.

SUMMARY

29. Exercise band training – hip abduction side to side

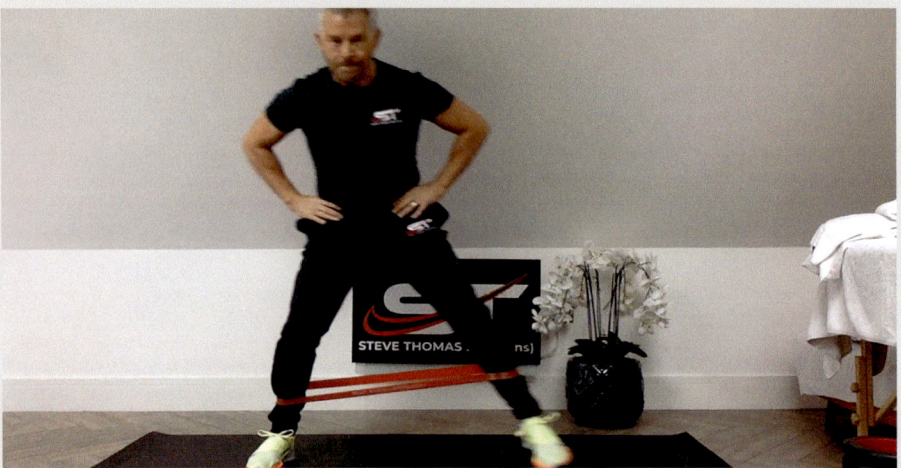

Place strong band around your ankles – step to one side – repeat multiple times leading with the same leg – change directions and repeat with other leg leading, until fatigue.

30. Static stretching – lying hamstring stretch

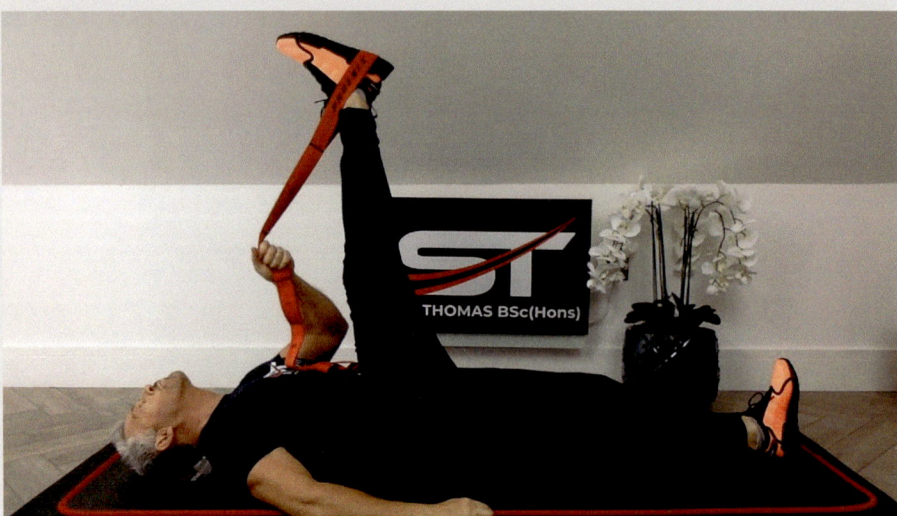

Lie on your back – place band around foot near heel (*do not place near toes*) – relax foot, point toes – pull leg into strong hamstring stretch – hold stationary for one to three minutes – repeat opposite leg.

SUMMARY

This example training routine highlights the variety of exercises, the positions, stretches, mobility movements, strength, speed, agility, flexibility, stamina/endurance, isolation and compound exercises that underpin my methods. It will teach you to understand and respect your entire musculoskeletal system.

The background research, the thought, the planning, the testing, the experimentation and the 100,000 one-to-one personal training sessions have all now been completed. It looks intricate, detailed and complex – because it is.

These 30 vital components and the intricate exercise 'jigsaw' or spreadsheet have taken nearly 40 years to develop, refine and structure into safe, comprehensive, productive routines that really do work for **everyone**. Yes, one system really does fit all – it fits **you** – so please understand and believe in the variety, balance and combination of these 30 components, and they will repay you handsomely.

For a comprehensive look at all my routines please visit the-father-figure-of-fitness.com. Remember that the research, experimentation, planning and testing of these routines have been done; your job now is to execute them correctly and consistently.

Remember also that the magic is in the detail – doing and feeling all these exercises and achieving the correct intensity is key. Detail and quality are everything. Exercise following my Top Tips and you will flourish like never before.

My **top tips** and ten **Golden Rules** follow.

My top tips

Golden Rule 1 – understand you

Your exercise routine must be about **you**. You must develop a comprehensive understanding of you by learning about you.

You are unique and you must understand what makes you unique. You have strengths but – please trust me – you also have your weaknesses, and you **must** acknowledge and address them.

Please don't just follow what others do – do what is necessary for **your** body.

Golden Rule 2 – understand biomechanics

Human biomechanics is the scientific understanding of the physical you: the way your musculoskeletal system works, how your brain, nerves, muscles, bones and joints all work together to determine **your** posture and movement.

Analysing **your** biomechanics is the key to understanding how your feet, ankles, knees, hips, pelvis, spine, head, neck and shoulders function, and this underpins the exercise routine that you should do.

Golden Rule 3 – analyse your leg length

Understanding and analysing your leg length is the first step in understanding how you stand, walk, jog, run and move.

Please understand that the vast majority of individuals have some leg length discrepancies that **must** be understood and addressed. Refer to chapter 5 to find out how to measure your leg length.

Golden Rule 4 – slow-motion video analysis

To understand your biomechanics, you must undertake slow-motion video analysis of your stance, walking and running (front, back and side view).

Standing and movement analysis using the naked eye may highlight any acute irregularities in your movement patterns, but it is the small deviations – the small nuances of your movement patterns – that are so important to analyse, understand and address and make your exercise routines bespoke for you.

Slow-motion video will enlighten you about **your** unique kinetic chain and your movement patterns. You can study how your feet influence your ankle movements, which in turn influence and dictate your knee movements, your hip movements, your pelvic movements, your spinal movements and your head, neck and shoulder movements.

This analysis will highlight and expose your mechanical weaknesses and uncover issues that otherwise you would never know existed. Please remember that we **all** have some deviation (however small), some mechanical weaknesses that we simply cannot ignore.

Please read how to take video footage in chapter 7.

Golden Rule 5 – safeguard your musculoskeletal system

I can assure you that you do have physical, structural, and musculoskeletal inefficiencies that require constant attention. Looking after your skeleton, your muscles, your bones and your joints is essential, regardless of your age, height, weight, fitness levels and experience, and is essential irrespective of your goals and ambitions.

Incorporating feet, ankle, knee, hip, pelvis, spine, neck and shoulder pre-habilitation and rehabilitation exercises, with extra emphasis on your hamstring muscles, your gluteal muscles and your spinal mobility exercises, will allow your musculoskeletal system to flourish, rather than holding you back.

Look after your physical body and it will repay you in kind.

Golden Rule 6 – variety

Variety of exercise and movement is really at the core of my 100,000 exercise system. Understanding not only our ancestors but the science of human movement dictates that you need variety in isolation exercises, variety in fluid compound movements and variety in joint range of movement stretches and exercises that constantly test out your body and keep it 'guessing'. This

MY TOP TIPS

ensures that it will continually adapt and progress, producing the fastest results possible.

This is why each of my exercise programmes has 30 different vital components that supply the constant variety of stimulation that the human body thrives on.

Golden Rule 7 – understand proprioception

Understanding the concept and importance of developing **your** proprioceptive ability is crucial if you want to master your craft.

During your muscular exercises you **must** *close your eyes, stop counting numbers* and learn to *focus, find, feel and fatigue* your muscles.

This proprioceptive 'feeling' of your movements – the experiencing of your muscles and movements – is imperative if you want to maximise **your** results.

Golden Rule 8 – be consistent, realistic and dedicated

We all live in a modern world in which impatience is everywhere. Given the correct quality, balance and diversity of exercise, your body will repay you handsomely if you exercise or train with precision, quality, variety and consistency.

Set realistic goals, be dedicated and be patient, and your body will respond like never before.

Golden Rule 9 – rest

Please be aware that many of your body's results are gained during your rest periods. This is simply how your body works and how your muscles adapt and progress.

Overtraining is a much bigger problem globally than one would expect. You must exercise with precision, detail, enthusiasm and intensity, but please respect your body's need to rest and recuperate.

MY TOP TIPS

Golden Rule 10 – use this mantra

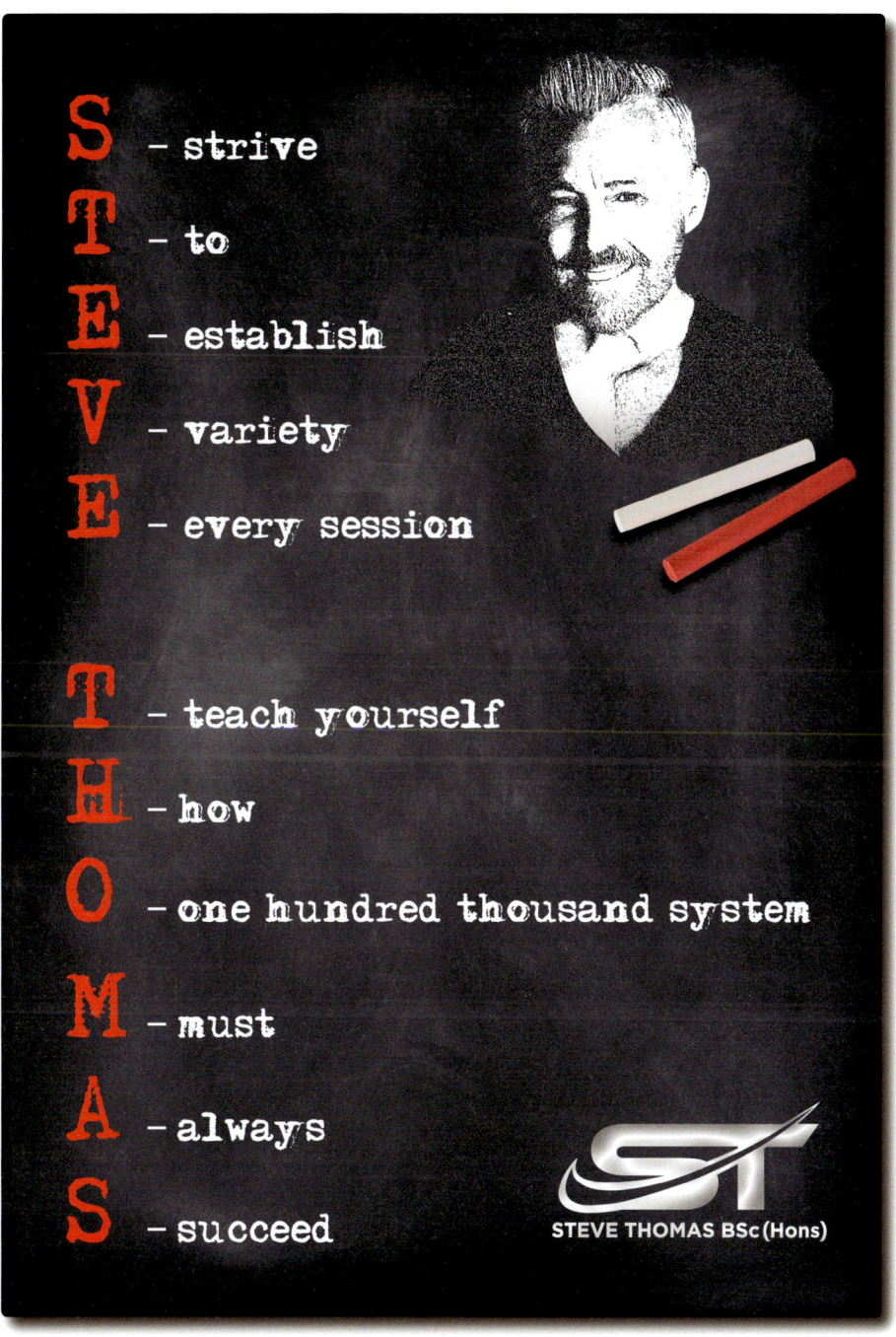

Conclusion

The human body is quite majestic in its complexity, and understanding how each and every individual should exercise safely and productively requires a diversity of information, advice and instruction.

My 37 years of experience have thrown up almost every scenario imaginable – beginners, elite athletes, old, young, athletic, not so athletic, underweight, overweight, fast responders, slow responders, those that are well coordinated and those that are not.

I have seen the results of good and bad training. I have worked with every kind of injury, surgery, pre-habilitation and rehabilitation patients, over- and under-enthusiastic clients and utilised and experimented with every known exercise and exercise routine ever established. As a result, every single minute of every single 100,000 one-to-one personal training session that I have completed has contributed in some way to my exercise system.

Establishing the world's most comprehensive system that **every** single one of us should follow has therefore been very complex and has covered many different aspects, all of which have tremendous value.

I have established that there are 30 vital components that we **all** need to understand and adhere to. Embrace these vital components and follow my **Top Tips** and ten **Golden Rules** and you will change the way you train for ever, releasing your body and allowing it to flourish like never before.

So let me be your personal trainer, let my knowledge and experience guide **you** to a better **you**.

This book has been written from the heart, from a lifelong ambition to bring science into exercise and from a long career seeking and developing an exercise system to set up the future of exercise.

This 100,000 system is my honest and heartfelt attempt to change the world of exercise. It's a campaign for change, a campaign to bring the science and medical world closer to the personal training world and it's a campaign to establish medical recognition for sport science and sports medicine graduates.

It's a campaign for a fitter, healthier society; a campaign for parents, teachers, doctors, youngsters and every other age group; a campaign to show the power of exercise.

But mostly it is a thank-you to my industry – an industry that has given me a great life – and it has mainly been written for **you**.

Please join my campaign and spread the word.

I am Steve Thomas, and *I am the father figure of fitness*.

Acknowledgements

This book has been a career-long ambition. It's a heartfelt, honest attempt to change the world of exercise. It's also a thank-you to an industry that has given me a wonderful life, to every one of my clients and especially to those that have become great friends and contributed to this book. It's a thank-you to Alan McQueen for his continued support. It's a thank-you to my family, my stepdaughter Sophie, my son-in-law Dale, grandchildren Amelia and Alfred and brothers Jeff and Mike for their support and belief, and it's a very special thank-you to my amazing wife Nikki for her love, patience, support and unconditional belief and encouragement both in me and in the writing of this book. Thank you, my darling.

I want to dedicate this book to my very special parents. They are no longer with us but remain in my heart every single minute of every single day. Their unconditional love provided me with the platform and freedom to dream and build a successful career. They will never be forgotten. Thank you, Mum and Dad.